FACT #1
The vast majority of victims endure
back pain unnecessarily.

FACT #2
There is no such thing as a slipped disc.

FACT #3
Fewer than 5% of all people with back pain
are likely to benefit from surgery.

In his clear, straightforward book, Hamilton Hall, M.D. debunks the numerous myths surrounding back problems. As a professor of surgery and Director of the Spine Service at the Orthopedic and Arthritic Hospital in Toronto, Dr. Hall is well qualified to do so. Dr. Hall is a member of the Canadian Orthopedic Association, the North American Spine Society, and the International Society for the Study of the Lumbar Spine. He founded the highly acclaimed Canadian Back Institute, an organization designed to educate backache victims in self-help methods of back care. The Back Institute is the largest centrally coordinated group of spine clinics in Canada.

THE NEW BACK DOCTOR

The Program for Lifetime Relief from Back Pain

Hamilton Hall, M.D.

Illustrated by Margot Mackay,
ANSCA, BSc AAM

SEAL BOOKS
McClelland-Bantam, Inc.
Toronto

Originally published as:
THE BACK DOCTOR
LIFETIME RELIEF FOR YOUR ACHING BACK

A Seal Book / published by arrangement with Macmillan of Canada

PUBLISHING HISTORY
Macmillan of Canada edition published September 1980
A selection of Literary Guild, Spring 1981
Seal edition / April 1982
Seal revised edition / January 1995
Reprinted June 1995

Illustrations by Margot Mackay, B.Sc. A.A.M., Department of Art as Applied to Medicine, University of Toronto

ISBN 0-7704-2619-0

PRINTED IN CANADA

UNI   20 19 18 17 16

Contents

Illustrations

Introduction

One evening not long ago, I was waiting to deliver some after-dinner remarks on the nature of back pain to an audience concerned with accident prevention. I found myself seated at the head table next to an expert in industrial safety.

My dinner companion wasn't a doctor but he had acquired a good deal of knowledge about industrial back injuries. He told me that he had heard me speak before and had enjoyed my comments on the misconceptions many people have about their backs. But he was curious about some of my remarks.

"You aren't going to tell them there's no such thing as a slipped disc?" he asked.

I replied that I would.

"But," he said, "don't you get into trouble with your colleagues, going around saying things like that?"

At that moment I realized that this safety expert was harboring his own misconception — that I was a squealer on my own profession, a sort of medical stool pigeon who was revealing secret truths about the human back.

That incident, described in the Introduction to the original *Back Doctor*, took place nearly twenty years ago. So much has happened to back care since then — so many advances, so much new technology — and yet the problem remains. Back pain is still the major source of recurring disability under the age of forty-five. It costs the North American economy more than $50 billion a year in reduced productivity, replacement costs, compensation payments, and medical expenses. Back pain still strikes eight out of every ten of us at some time in our adult life and, for an unfortunate minority, it becomes a lifelong problem.

With newer perspectives and altered attitudes, I marvel that the basic message of *The Back Doctor* remains so relevant. Its approach and most of its practical advice are as necessary today as they were when I prepared the first manuscript. The "slipped disc" is just as real as it was when I entered the field. Back pain is not a disease; it is a human condition. Back pain does not demand a cure; it demands control. Understanding the problem is the first step, and that understanding has grown enormously. What was intuition is now supported with fact; theory has become practice. But there is so much more to know.

My twenty years with the Canadian Back Institute have taught me a great deal and I am indebted to all the physiotherapists and kinesiologists who have patiently demonstrated their expertise. I recognize how difficult it is to impart skill in pain control and confidence in the potential for recovery to someone in the grips of an excruciating back pain attack. I realize how frustrating it is to promote the idea of regular exercise to someone who has never even tried. And I have learned what a daunting task it is to persuade anyone to return to activity while the pain lingers on.

Special thanks to Tony Melles, senior physiotherapist and executive director of the Canadian Back Institute, for all the hours we have spent exchanging ideas and refining the concepts presented in my first book and elaborated here. It was Tony who showed me how rapidly mechanical back pain can be eliminated with posture correction and early movement. His recurring analogies of the light switch — "You should be able to turn the pain on and off" — and the cut finger — "Protect the cut while it heals, then start moving again" — have become part of my litany for common backache. He is also responsible for my clear separation between the necessary "strain" pain of recovering function in tight tissue and the unwanted recurrence of the "typical" pain that initially marked the problem.

I still ask only ten minutes a day for your back care program, but now I recommend that the time be spread throughout your waking hours to achieve lasting pain control.

If I could do it all again and today write *The Back Doctor* for the first time, I would make only one fundamental change. But it is such an important alteration that, at the risk of confusing the tens of thousands of readers who have already studied my work, I am making it now. Mechanical back pain begins with the disc. We have gained a clearer picture of its loss of normal function and the cascade effect this has on the other components of the spine. It may not be the only source of pain, but it is almost always the first site of trouble. For this reason, I will designate disc-related complaints as Pattern One. Incidentally, this is also the most common pattern of pain I am called upon to treat — another good reason to put it first. Because changes in the small spinal joints typically result from a loss of resilience in the discs and are therefore a secondary phenomenon, I will designate small joint problems as Pattern Two. Instead of my three types of back pain, I now acknowledge four. In addition to reversing the order of the first two, I am adding a second pattern of leg-dominant pain to accompany Pattern Three, the pain of acute nerve compression I described in the first book. Pattern Four is leg pain rapidly produced by activity and rapidly relieved by rest and posture change.

The term "Pattern" replaces "Type" for an important reason. It is the pattern of typical back pain, rather than the possible anatomical location of the problem, that determines treatment. Although there is general consensus about the causes of each pattern, some disagreement remains. Rather than cloud the issue by mixing the observable and easily recognizable with disputed theories about probable cause, I have emphasized those elements that can be identified by anyone who reads this book. It is, after all, your ability to select your own typical pattern of pain from the examples in these pages that will enable you to take control.

I have expanded the section on pain-focused behavior. All pain is real, but not all back pain begins in the back. As difficult as it is to accept, the amount of pain is not a measure of the seriousness of the problem. When pain dominates your life, nothing is the same and, until you can confront the real villain, there can be no lasting recovery. Dealing with the four patterns of mechanical back pain begins with recognition. Dealing with pain behavior is no different. It's difficult to fight what you cannot see. Finding yourself in a description of the pain-focused individual should not be the end of the story. It can be the first step to regaining control of your life.

Some things have changed in twenty years. Investigative techniques such as epidural venograms and the epiduragram mentioned in the original *Back Doctor* have disappeared. Tomography is almost never used, and the myelogram is being eliminated. Magnetic resonance imaging (MRI) has taken the place of computerized axial tomography (CT) as the investigation of last resort. New outpatient surgical techniques deal with disc herniations through half-inch (1 cm) incisions. And non-surgical care has evolved into a more precise and reproducible form. Even limited periods of bed rest are being abandoned in favor of exercise and activation. Specific exercises provide rapid pain control and simple posture correction offers lasting relief.

I have developed a more balanced view, perhaps the result of examining more than thirty thousand patients with neck and low back pain. *The New Back Doctor* is my attempt to translate what I have learned of low back pain into the vocabulary of the average back pain sufferer. It reflects my belief in the value of exercises that arch the spine backwards as well as forwards; of proper posture and the maintenance of a neutral curve in the low back to promote rapid pain control, and of the need to develop a carefully structured personal program that can be assimilated into an unstructured lifestyle.

This book marks my first major effort without the guidance and support of my friend and teacher Hal Tennant. His spirit lives on in these pages, and his gentle reminder to "just say what you mean" is a challenge never forgotten.

Nothing works for everyone, but everyone can find something that works. Since 1974 that philosophy has helped the Canadian Back Institute grow from a series of educational lectures to the largest centrally coordinated group of back care clinics in Canada. CBI is close to seeing more patients in a year than I have seen in a lifetime of practice. With the aid of computerized data collection and a standardized outcome review, the clinics are poised to research the question of low back pain in ways never before possible.

The New Back Doctor offers you an opportunity to know more about your back and with that knowledge a chance to solve your own problem. It is not a self-help book as much as a field guide to the recognition of common patterns of back pain. Knowing their habits and habitats will make their sudden appearance less frightening and their rapid departure more likely.

I want to put you in charge, to eliminate your dependence on anyone or anything. Back pain creates a sense of helplessness only when you lack the ability to fight back. Providing you with the knowledge and skill to stop your pain today and control it tomorrow is what this book is all about.

Hamilton Hall, MD, FRCSC
Toronto, May 1994

attempt to "just say what you mean" is accordingly
never forgotten.

Nothing works the same way, but every one has had
schooling that works. Since 1983, that philosophy has
helped drag Canadian back management from a review of
abnormal structure to the largest carefully orchestrated
group of back-care clinics in Canada. CBI's close to seeing
its crew patients treated, that I have such in a lifetime
of practice. With the aid of computerized data analysis
and a standardized outcome review, the lines are poised
to research the question of how best pain matters most
and by how little.

YOU, As Back Doctor, offers you an opportunity to
get more in-depth with back and with that knowledge, a
chance to measure your own problem. It is not a self-help
book as much as a field guide to the recognition of common problems of back pain. You who have held backs and
families will make their studied appearance here, helping
you and them to recognize more health.

I hope to put you in charge to eliminate your expectations on abroad, recognizing that in one stroke a sense
of helplessness only works to slack the desire to fight
back. Providing you with the knowledge and skill to win
your own battle and control is return are is what this
book is all about.

Hamilton Hall, MD, FRCSC
Toronto, May 199?

1 *The Things a Back Doctor Hears*

Every year, several thousand men and women parade through my office, one by one, complaining of back pain. That in itself is hardly surprising. As an orthopedic surgeon — a bone-and-joint doctor — I specialize in helping people with back problems. And, like most people who work hard at a subject they know, I've had my share of successes.

The remarkable thing about my work, though, is the amount of time I have to spend educating people about their own spines. Don't misunderstand me. My patients are intelligent people. In most respects, including the fact that they suffer from back pain, they're quite typical of the population at large. But, also typically, they have absorbed an appalling amount of misinformation about the human back. After listening to these people talk about their backs, day after day, year after year, I am convinced that no other part of the human body — not the brain, not the sex organs, not even the heart with all its symbolic mystique — has given rise to so many misconceptions, so much silly folklore, and so many unwarranted fears.

I've discovered that the human back is regarded as such an enigma that people concerned with back problems often abandon all common sense and whatever knowledge they do possess of physiology. They apply peculiar tests and rules they would never dream of applying to other parts of their bodies.

It's all so self-defeating.

There is such a thing, of course, as harmless superstition, even when it applies to your back. Remember that old rhyme we used to recite as kids whenever we walked along a concrete sidewalk? "Step on a crack — break your mother's back!" Some of the commonest beliefs adults have about their backs are just as absurd as that children's rhyme. But they are far from harmless. Misinformation encourages countless numbers of people to behave self-destructively. They endure back pain unnecessarily. They undergo treatments and exercises that are needlessly painful and in some cases useless. And meanwhile they forgo many satisfying activities — golf, gardening, or sex — that they could be enjoying.

If that description fits your situation, this book is meant for you. It will tell you the things I tell my patients, and more — everything you need to know about your back: how it's put together, how it works, why it sometimes becomes painful, and how you can control or even eliminate that pain.

It is important, first of all, to rid yourself of any false notions you may have about your back. Let's begin by looking at the beliefs I hear voiced, day after day, by new patients.

"The human back is a very special part of the body."

Certainly your back is special in the sense that it's important. But so are your brain, your heart, your liver, and many of your other organs. Your back is not unique. In fact its parts are remarkably similar to those found elsewhere in your body: its bones have an internal structure like a honeycomb — just as your heel bones have. It has small joints that are like the joints in your fingers. Its discs are quite similar to a joint you have in the front of your pelvis. Its muscles are much like the muscles in your thighs. Its ligaments resemble the ligaments in your ankles. Even the tunnel in each vertebra, through which your spinal cord passes, isn't all that different from the openings in the backs of your eye sockets, through which the optic nerves enter the brain.

"My back is a hopelessly confusing piece of anatomy with problems so complex they are impossible to diagnose."

If you happen to share that belief, I'd like to ask you why. Is your back a mystery to you because you can't get a good look at it? Or does it frighten you because it has parts with strange names like cervical vertebrae and sacrum and coccyx? Perhaps you are bewildered by diagrams you've seen of the human back, with its intricate array of bones and muscles and ligaments and nerves. Or did a doctor alarm you by saying he wasn't sure what was causing your pain?

Suppose I told you that I own a mysterious and complex machine called an automobile. It has thousands of parts, including many I've never seen. A lot of these parts have strange names — like carburetor and cylinder head and alternator. Could I convince you, on the evidence, that this mysterious machine of mine is capable of breakdowns that can baffle the best minds in the automotive world?

Hardly. You would rightly point out that whatever might go wrong with my car, all I need is either a skilled mechanic or a good repair manual and the right tools. You might agree that the repairs could be expensive and time-consuming. But you would continue to insist that my "mystery machine" couldn't possibly be too complicated for diagnosis by a competent repairman.

Neither is your back.

"My back is one of the most fragile parts of my body."

Do you think so? Let me tell you about an airline accident that proved just the opposite.

At eight o'clock on the morning of Monday, June 26, 1978, Air Canada Flight 189, a DC-9 jetliner bound for Winnipeg, began its takeoff from Toronto International Airport. Flight 189 never got off the ground. As it reached a speed of 120 miles an hour, the plane skidded off the runway and plunged 50 feet (15 m) into a ravine. Fifty feet is a long drop, equivalent to driving your car off the roof of a five-story building.

The DC-9 carried 107 people — passengers and crew. All were wearing seat belts. As the plane hit the bottom of the ravine, they were thrown violently forward. The impact of the crash was estimated later at 25 to 30 g — four to five times the gravitational force astronauts experience during a launching. Pinned into place by the belts around their midsections, the plane's occupants were literally folded in half. The strain on their backs was tremendous. Yet fewer than half the people aboard that plane suffered back injuries. Make no mistake about it, this was a serious accident. Two passengers died (though not from spinal injuries) and many others, subjected to an enormous force while restrained by their seat belts, suffered serious injuries to their backs. My point, however, is that in spite of those forces, the majority of the people aboard survived without back injuries of any kind. If our backs were as fragile as many of my patients suppose, nobody could have come away from Flight 189 without serious spinal damage.

Or consider the case of the apprehensive adulterer. Mr. X became a patient of mine immediately after undergoing a disastrous and terrifying experience. He had developed a passion for a certain woman who, unfortunately for him, was married to someone else. One night, the classic confrontation occurred. The amorous couple was discovered together in her sixth-floor apartment. Whether Mr. X jumped or was pushed I never learned, but, either way, he tumbled from the sixth-floor balcony, landing on his feet on the roof of a neighboring two-story house. You can imagine how the impact was transmitted up through his body. When I examined him in the emergency room, I found Mr. X had broken both heels and both legs and had suffered various internal and head injuries. And yet there was nothing wrong with his spine.

"I've been told I have a slipped disc. Can you put it back into place for me?"

You may find this hard to believe, but there is no such thing as a slipped disc. I know you've heard the expression dozens of times, and even your own doctor may have used it. If so, he didn't intend to convey the impression it gave you. Most people know they have discs between their vertebrae. They imagine a disc to be something like a poker chip — thin, hard, and slippery, and thus capable of popping easily out of position. When this happens, they think they need a professional — a chiropractor, a physiotherapist, or a doctor like me — to pop it back into place for them. In reality, discs never slip out of place. They bulge.

We'll be going into more detail about discs in a later chapter, but for the moment forget about the poker-chip image. Think, instead, of a tap washer — that little rubber doughnut that seals off the flow of water in a faucet. If you've ever changed a washer, you will have noticed that when you fasten it down tight, the washer bulges slightly. That's roughly what happens whenever there's pressure on a disc in your spine. When a disc bulges far enough to come into contact with a nerve — an uncommon occurrence, incidentally — the condition is often referred to as a slipped disc. But I think it's a pity the term ever came into use, and I wish people, especially doctors, would stop using it. It conjures up an image that is false and frightening.

"I could tell the instant my back went out — I heard it crack."
Like the slipped disc, the notion of a person's back "going out" is part of modern folklore. Comedian George Burns, always ready with a gag based on his advancing years, once declared: "At my age, my back goes out more often than I do." When someone tells me his back has "gone out," the expression makes me want to ask, "Where did it go? Did it stay out all night, or did it come tiptoeing back around 2 a.m. with some lame excuse about having to sit up with a sick friend?"

Just as it is erroneous to describe a disc as having "slipped," it is wrong to describe a spine as having "gone out." It is true that under certain circumstances you may hear a cracking sound in your spine. That sound is the same as the one that is heard when a person cracks his or her knuckles. In the joints of your fingers and in your spinal joints you have nitrogen in solution, under pressure. If you pull suddenly on your finger, you decrease the pressure in the joint. This causes the nitrogen to come out of solution and turn temporarily from liquid to gas in much the same way that champagne goes "pop" when you uncork the bottle. Now, to many people, the act of cracking the knuckle is as offensive as belching at the dinner table. But it's not harmful. And just as nobody ever pulled a finger off while cracking his knuckles, nobody ever "threw his back out," even though it may have sounded like it.

If you hear a cracking sound when you're having your spine manipulated by a physiotherapist or a chiropractor, you may believe that one or several vertebrae have been snapped back into place. But the truth is that your back has never really been "out." The bones of your back are linked by discs and small joints. The bones can move in relation to each other the same way the bones in your arms or legs do. But they remain solidly connected and in the correct alignment. Like your arms or legs, your back has great flexibility, but the moving parts maintain exactly the correct position. If, after your back makes a cracking sound, you suffer pain or experience relief, there are other reasons why.

"My back hurts. Do you suppose it's arthritis?"

Could be. But that doesn't explain what's causing the pain. The first syllable of "arthritis" comes from the Greek word for joint. The suffix "-itis" means an inflammation, which is a condition, not a disease. Inflammation is the body's response to a variety of problems, from chemical irritation to physical injury. It is the release of a number of substances, including white blood cells, designed to promote healing and speed repair. Every time you add "-itis" to a body part, you are describing this process. Tendinitis, tonsillitis, and appendicitis are all examples of local inflammation.

Arthritis, then, is simply an inflamed joint.

Suppose you noticed I had inflamed eyes, commonly called bloodshot eyes but technically referred to as conjunctivitis. You would realize instantly that it was a condition, not a disease in itself, and you might ask whether it was the result of an accident or an illness, or perhaps evidence of a hangover. What you might not realize is that I could also suffer an inflamed or "bloodshot" condition in almost any joint of my body. I could get a "bloodshot" or inflamed toe joint by stubbing my toe while walking barefoot on a rocky beach. Or I might get the same condition in one of my spinal joints as a result of an accident, disease, or — commonest of all — plain, old-fashioned wear. Wherever my inflamed joint might be located, it would properly be referred to as arthritis.

Patients often tell me their back pain is caused by "arthritis". To them it is a disease, one that is likely to spread to other joints beyond the spine. For most people the word "arthritis," a condition, is synonymous with "rheumatoid arthritis," a disease. And that's not the case. Back pain from ordinary wear in the small spinal joints probably affects thirty percent of the adult population and it's not a disease at all.

Now that you understand the words, you understand why patients who believe they have "arthritis of the spine" are relieved when I tell them that what they really have is "inflammation of the small spinal joints." It is, of course, exactly the same thing, but it sounds so much safer.

Once you understand that arthritis is a condition that could have any one of several causes, you realize there is no such thing as a single cure for it. More important, you appreciate that arthritis, as a word, is really nothing to fear. And as a condition, it may be no more serious than a bloodshot eye or a stubbed toe.

"I don't dare work in the garden (play tennis, have sex) for fear of injuring my back."

I must say I sympathize with people who feel that way. What they should understand, however, is that there is an important difference between pain and injury. Tending your tulips may cause pain in your back, but it won't cause injury. As we've already seen, your back can stand a lot of abuse without suffering actual damage. Often you'll feel pain simply because you are using muscles in some unaccustomed way, or pushing them beyond their normal limits. To test this principle for yourself, pick up a heavy book and hold it in one hand at arm's length. Within a few minutes your arm muscles will begin to complain. Later the pain will become intense. And yet you won't damage your arm. At the most, you'll have sore arm muscles for a while. But so what? We've all experienced muscular soreness — from painting a ceiling, or wheeling topsoil for the lawn, or riding horseback, especially if it's for the first time. Without suffering bruises or other injuries, we can incur pain, either at the time or later, or both.

The same principle applies to your back, even if it has been sore in the past. No normal activities, such as lobbing a tennis ball, swinging a golf club, or mowing the lawn, will damage your back. But they may cause pain. It may be more than muscular pain; it may even be acute and severe pain resulting from stress on your discs or spinal joints. But it won't cause damage. And only you can decide whether the activity provides enjoyment that's worth the price of the pain.

Whenever you choose to endure a certain amount of pain in return for a pleasurable experience, you're making a trade-off. I will have more to say about trade-offs in a later chapter. Meanwhile, start getting used to the idea that even an acutely painful activity won't damage your back. "Hurt" is not the same as "harm."

"I don't remember ever injuring my back, but I must have or it wouldn't be hurting — right?"

Wrong. Many people are surprised to learn that almost two-thirds of back attacks begin for no immediate reason at all. In some circumstances, when filing an insurance claim, for example, a specific cause must be listed. But that doesn't mean one necessarily exists. And when back injury is a factor, the pain begins within hours of the event. Remember, your back is not unique, and what happens here is no different than what happens in the rest of your body. No sensible person would accept the idea of being able to suffer a broken leg or a dislocated elbow without realizing until much later that some serious damage had occurred. Yet many people are willing to believe that the equivalent injury could happen to their spines without their knowing it.

Such is the mystique of the human back. And, like several other popular myths, it ignores the commonest cause of back pain: the ordinary wear that is a normal part of living and growing older.

"It's an old childhood injury, but it hasn't bothered me for years — until now."

Not long ago, a woman of twenty-eight came to see me about a pain in her back. She had already decided what had caused her problem. At the age of five she fell off a porch and hurt her back. I asked her how often she'd had back pain during the twenty-three years since her accident. "Never," she said, "until just last week."

This "childhood injury" theory has no basis in medical experience, and yet I can understand why people are ready to believe it. If you have back pain, it's natural to assume you've been injured. Most people try to pin down the "when" and the "how." They have no trouble dredging up a recollection of some plausible-sounding incident. All of us have had childhood accidents or misadventures that seemed, and perhaps were, quite serious at the time: a fall off a bicycle or a garage roof; an accident in a too-shallow swimming pool; a bodily collision on a playing field. If an old injury has bothered you, off and on, for years, then it may in fact have some relationship to a present pain. But there is no such thing as a serious bone or joint injury lying dormant for years and then suddenly flaring up. That may seem to have happened to your back, but in reality your present pain must have some other cause.

"It must be really serious — the pain is unbearable."

Here's another fact you may find hard to believe: there is little relationship between the seriousness of a back problem and the amount of pain it causes. Some serious ailments cause only mild pain. Conversely, you can suffer severe pain from a short-lived condition that is no threat to your health. The condition called wry neck is a good example. Wry neck is a form of muscle spasm that can cause excruciating pain to shoot up and down your neck with the slightest turning of your head. Yet it causes no damage, it's usually gone in a few days, and it may never recur.

"It's bad enough having the pain in my back, but I'm afraid it will spread to the rest of my body and leave me paralyzed."

That would be a terrifying prospect if it were real. Perhaps you are among those who imagine your back problem to be an insidious disease that is coursing up and down your spine, threatening to spread to your arms and legs. Fortunately, that isn't what back pain is all about. Most back conditions cause some pain to be relayed into the legs. But the cause of your pain is almost certain to be located in one small part of your spine, probably in a disc or in one of the small joints we call facet (rhymes with cassette) joints. In all likelihood it's a mechanical problem, comparable to a worn or damaged engine part. The wear will interfere with normal function and in the back this means pain. A little extra load will shift to nearby discs and joints, but the mechanical failure won't spread like some contagious disease. On the contrary, with proper care and exercise, it will probably repair itself and the pain will go away.

"I'm only thirty-six and my back is so bad already I'm sure it will deteriorate by the time I'm sixty."

Your prospects are probably much better than you think. Statistically, back pain is less frequent in old age. I often compare a patient's spine to a machine, to illustrate how wear can impair efficient function. But, unlike an old car, your back has the capability of repairing itself, and eventually this is what happens to the majority of people who have common backache during middle age. The peak incidence of mechanical back pain is in the early forties, although the problem can begin as early as the late teens. Backache tends to be episodic, recurring throughout life with the frequency increasing in the middle years. Women appear to have a second period of increased trouble in their late fifties, but for both men and women the incidence of attacks decreases with age. If you live long enough, you will outlive your back pain. Of course, there's no guarantee that you will be among those who benefit from natural mending, but the statistics are definitely on your side. This, incidentally, is one reason why backache is such an economic and social problem: it strikes more often during people's working years, not after retirement.

The natural healing process takes years and is accompanied by joint stiffness and loss of height. Certainly a seventy-year-old doesn't have the spinal flexibility of a teenager. But, typically, the back pain is gone and the spine has retained enough strength and movement to satisfy the most active senior citizen. I recall two participants in one of my back education classes, a mother and her daughter. The daughter was in her mid-sixties; her mother was eighty-five. The daughter was there because she had a back problem. Her mother just came along for company. "I used to have back trouble when I was her age," the mother explained, "but now it's all better."

I am not suggesting that back pain is unknown in old age. Some elderly people do suffer from it. But they are a minority, and their backs are rarely afflicted by the mechanical conditions I am discussing throughout this book. In elderly people, backache is more often related to a bony narrowing of the central canal through which the nerves travel or to bony conditions such as osteoporosis, a weakening of the bones through a loss of normal structure that renders the vertebrae more vulnerable to fracture. (This and other rarer causes of backache are described in Chapter Five.)

"My husband says I'm just imagining the pain, and I'm beginning to wonder if he's right."

All pain is real. If you feel pain, there is pain. You are not "just imagining the whole thing." But it is also true that your emotions can add to your discomfort or even bring on an attack of pain. Once you have experienced back pain, it is impossible not to have an emotional response to it. The very fact that you dread and fear it can make the pain worse than it would otherwise be.

Your emotions can also cause a pain attack, through their relationship with body tension. We all know that when we experience certain emotions, the muscles in our bodies become tense. That happens to all of us whether we have back problems or not; in moments of stress, our muscles tighten up, especially in our necks and along our spines. It's no wonder that supervisor who gets you so upset is a real "pain in the neck." If you happen to have worn discs or joints in your spine, the muscular tension that is associated with emotion puts pressure on these areas and that causes even more pain.

However your emotions are related to your back pain, it's incorrect and unfair to suggest that "it's just your imagination."

"My back will always be painful until I find exactly the right mattress (office chair, car seat)."

Unlike most misconceptions I hear from my patients, this one usually develops after the person has learned a bit about back care, such as the best positions for standing, sitting, and sleeping. According to the old expression, a little learning can be a dangerous thing; but I've found that with back patients it's usually just boring or silly.

One of my patients is a man who brings his car-seat problem into my office. We go over it together. Should it be tilted five degrees or only three? I try to tell him he ought to arrange it in whatever way is most comfortable. But that's not enough for him: he always insists on pinning me down to an exact number. So I may tell him to make it six and a half degrees or fourteen degrees, depending on the mood I happen to be in that morning.

Mr. Car Seat is forever buying and selling cars, always according to his current notion of seat comfort. Whatever make or model he has chosen, he jams magazines under the driver's seat. He believes that, as his back doctor, I should decide whether he's likely to be more comfortable with *Time* or with *Playboy*. Obviously the man is obsessed. But I can't tell him the whole thing is a figment of his imagination. Instead, I let him go through his routine. If he announces this week that an eight-degree tilt and three copies of *Sports Illustrated* under the seat are just right, I say, "Fine."

Who am I to argue? Having reviewed the latest literature in my field, I can tell you that medical science has yet to come up with the perfect car seat, the perfect office chair, or the perfect mattress. Some chairs and mattresses are better than others, but what's perfect for one person may be uncomfortable for another. And in any event, what you sit on or sleep on is far less important than the *way* you sit and the *way* you lie when you sleep. I hope, some day, to get that point across to Mr. Car Seat.

"If my back problem is serious, I expect I'll have to undergo surgery."

To almost every back patient I see, I explain two basic points about surgery. One is that fewer than two percent of all people with back pain are likely to benefit from surgery. About ninety-eight out of a hundred, including serious cases, are better off with some combination of physiotherapy, medication, exercise, and what we refer to as proper ADL — activities of daily living; that is, the proper positions when standing, sitting, lying in bed, and so on.

The second point is that surgery is no magic solution to any back problem. Surgery is the ultimate mechanical solution to a local mechanical difficulty. If the problem is located in one specific spot, if it is diagnosed properly, and if it does not respond to other forms of treatment —

all these ifs are important — then surgery may be the answer to your problem. But if the pain is originating from more than one point in your spine, or if the cause is not structural in nature, no surgeon can provide a solution with one swift, neat operation. He can't operate on pain; there must be a specific physical condition that can be corrected or improved by surgery.

When I have a patient who does need surgery, I always emphasize two other points, both of which follow from what I've just said. The first is that no matter how successful the operation is, your back will never be normal again; surgery creates scar tissue, which doesn't exist in a normal back. My second point is that even the most successful surgical operation is just one of several steps necessary to control the problem. If you are to undergo surgery, you must be prepared to make permanent changes in your lifestyle after the operation, doing the exercises and adopting the daily postural habits that will maintain your back in good condition, free of pain.

Your function and your ability may return to normal, but your back never will.

"Other people may have back problems, but mine is unique."
We all like to think we're special. Ordinary ailments are for ordinary people. It nurtures our ego to believe that whatever ailment we have is rare in the annals of medicine. Without actually saying so, most of my patients feel that if they have to be ill, then, dammit, they're going to suffer from something unusual and dramatic.

I was given a vivid demonstration of this phenomenon by a class of twenty-five people, all of whom had back pain. At the time I spoke to them, these people already knew that the three commonest causes of back pain were disc trouble, wear in a facet joint, and a pinched nerve. They also knew that of those three causes, the pinched nerve is the least common, occurring in only about one case out of every ten. I asked the members of this group to tell me, by a show of hands, which of these causes they believed was responsible for their own back pain.

Put yourself in their place. How much sympathy could you expect if you announced at your next cocktail party, "My doctor says I have a worn facet joint?" Can't you just see people's eyes beginning to glaze over already? Now try this one, "Did you ever have a pinched nerve in your spine? Well, I have. . . ." Now there's a medical drama for you. It feels painful just to describe it.

By now, you can guess how my class of twenty-five people responded to my question. Even knowing how low the statistical chances were, every man and woman in that room thought that he or she had a pinched nerve. No one was willing to settle for just a little wear in a disc or joint. Their pain was too severe and their disability too profound to be caused by anything less than a damaged nerve. I knew otherwise. They were all my patients and I had examined them all, one by one, and none of them had a nerve problem. They had all simply picked the cause they considered the most spectacular.

"I've been to five other doctors with this problem, and not one of them told me what you have just been telling me now."

That may be true. But often a doctor tries to explain a back problem without managing to get his message across. Some doctors don't take the necessary time to explain. Others find it hard to express themselves without using a lot of medical jargon that their patients don't understand. Even when the doctor spells out the whole thing in plain English, the patient may be too bewildered or too fearful to absorb and remember the information.

I don't pretend to be a genius at doctor-patient communications. But I work at it. And I try to make sure my patients understand everything they ought to know about their backs — what's wrong and what needs to be done to make it right. Even so, I find myself dealing with patients at moments when they are too upset to appreciate what I'm telling them.

That's one reason why I believe this book should be helpful. A lot of the information here might not be new to you, but it might seem new simply because you can consider it calmly and appreciate it more readily than when you heard it from your doctor. Even if it seems familiar, it will reinforce what you already know and enlarge your understanding of your problem.

As you read through the chapters that follow, I hope you will adopt the techniques I suggest for preventing common backache. I hope you will acquire the self-confidence and ability to cope with any attack you cannot prevent. And I wish you the satisfaction of accepting trade-offs by which you tolerate some pain in exchange for the enjoyment of a favorite activity you once avoided.

Most of all, I hope that the information in the rest of this book will help you substitute knowledge for any fear you now feel toward your back pain and its cause. For, in eliminating that fear, you will eliminate much of the pain itself.

2   Bogeyman, Ping-Pong, and Other Diversions

How do people with back problems manage to pick up so much harmful information?

I can think of many ways. They listen to old wives' tales. They diagnose themselves incorrectly and exchange their erroneous findings with their friends. They misquote articles they've read. And in some instances, sad to say, they can cite their own doctors as the source of their false notions and unwarranted fears.

There's a double irony here. For one thing, doctors are supposedly reliable sources of medical information and advice. For another, few patients of any kind are more in need of clear and accurate information, both general and specific, than those who suffer from back pain.

Yet there are family practitioners and even specialists who speak loosely of "slipped discs" and backs that have "gone out," even though they know better. And there are family doctors and specialists too who avoid talking frankly to their patients and resort instead to evasion, innuendo, and incomprehensible jargon.

Why do some doctors behave this way?

In many instances, I'm sure, it's purely unintentional — simply a matter of their being less sensitive or less adept at interpersonal communication than they might be. In other instances, I believe, they resort to game-playing because they feel uneasy and unsure of themselves when confronted with back patients and their problems. Often their discomfort is obvious, even to laymen. Once, at a social gathering, I met a man who said he derived great satisfaction from taking his wife around to see doctor after doctor about her bad back. He explained that he hated medical people, and "I like to watch a doctor sweat."

Many family doctors are uneasy with back pain because they find it tricky to diagnose and unsatisfying to treat. Some specialists, on the other hand, find it a bore. To a surgeon whose passion is the operating room, back patients are chronic complainers whose conditions neither appeal to his mentality nor challenge his well-honed skills. A back problem cannot be diagnosed precisely the way, say, a fractured wrist can. The treatment a back needs will likely be non-surgical. The improvement it shows will require frequent observation and minute adjustments. And a cure is out of the question. All in all, the doctor who is dedicated exclusively to surgery sees back treatment as a thankless and unrewarding task.

Although I don't share that view, I can understand and sympathize with it. The conduct that results, however, is something else, since it has a seriously detrimental effect on many patients who deserve better. Such effects are evident among some of the people who visit the average medical clinic or private medical office.

If you have ever gone to a doctor to complain of back pain, you may recognize yourself as the patient in one, or several, of the following games.

Speaking Doctor

In my private life, I speak English, just as most of my patients do. In my professional life, however, I communicate with my colleagues in medical jargon — a language I call Doctor. Like the jargon of other occupations, Doctor has its place. But it doesn't belong in a doctor-patient consultation, such as this one:

PATIENT: Doctor, I have something wrong with my neck.
DOCTOR (examining): You have cervical spondylosis.
PATIENT (recoiling): Oh, my God!

What did the doctor actually say here? He used the term "cervical spondylosis." If the patient had had a Doctor-English dictionary at hand, she could have discovered that "cervical" refers to the neck, "spondyl" indicates the spine, and "-osis" means disease of or, more loosely, something wrong with. Hence, "cervical spondylosis" is simply Doctor for something wrong with (the spinal portion of) your neck.

When the exchange is rendered entirely in English, it comes out in this improbable form:

PATIENT: Doctor, I have something wrong with my neck.
DOCTOR (examining): You have something wrong with your neck.
PATIENT (recoiling): Oh, my God!

As you might suppose, this game can be played with any Doctor term referring to any part of the body. For example:

PATIENT: Doctor, look at this rash on my skin.
DOCTOR: Ah, a case of dermatosis! (Derma = skin; -osis = disorder)
PATIENT: And I thought it was only a rash!

As you can see, the Doctor language has the power among laymen to make even the most mundane diagnosis sound terribly profound, medically learned — and frightening. That's not really why doctors use it. They learn to speak Doctor in medical school because they can't practice medicine without it. By the time they graduate, they've been exposed to fifty thousand words of Doctor. And it's invaluable to them. It has precision. It's concise. And it's universally understood within the medical community.

A few doctors may speak Doctor to their patients to mask their own diagnostic weaknesses, but I believe the trouble usually begins when the doctor forgets that his patients understand only a few terms — words like stethoscope and tonsillectomy. Without intending to bewilder or frighten anyone, he may lapse completely into Doctor, using many expressions known only to medical people. Ironically, at that moment, he may be attempting to allay the patient's fears, as in, "This is only a contusion." Those are not necessarily reassuring words to someone who doesn't realize that a contusion is just a bruise.

The game of speaking Doctor is especially unfortunate when it's played with back patients, because their treatment depends for its success on their thorough understanding of what's causing their pain, what they can do about it, and why they needn't be afraid of it. If your doctor uses a term you don't understand, ask for a translation, and don't be intimidated by those ten-dollar words.

But even plain English, imprudently used, can frighten a back patient, as we see in this next game.

Bogeyman

In nearly a century of film-making, the creators of horror movies have proved that audiences can be frightened most by the unknown. We all react with greater terror when the Thing is still on the other side of the door. We've all watched horror movies where the monster's appearance was a letdown because its unseen presence beforehand was far scarier.

The underlying principle, of course, is simple: nothing we are told or shown is as frightening as what we can concoct in our own imaginations. The game I call Bogeyman is based on this principle, which, again, is often evoked unintentionally by doctors when they say things they don't really mean, or when they imply more than they intend to. Either way, there are usually four elements in this game, with only the first element — the doctor's statement — spoken aloud. The other elements consist of what the Bogeyman whispers to the patient, what the doctor actually meant, and what the patient needed to hear at that moment for his own information or reassurance.

In a family practitioner's office it might go this way:

THE DOCTOR SAYS:
I don't know what's causing your pain.

THE BOGEYMAN WHISPERS:
In other words, you have a mysterious disease — cancer maybe!

THE DOCTOR MEANT:
I know ordinary back pain when I see it, but in your case I can't pinpoint the exact cause or source.

THE PATIENT NEEDED TO HEAR:
I can't determine the exact source of your pain, but that's not important at the moment. The first thing to do is a few gentle stretches, which will probably make the pain go away.

In a surgeon's office, a Bogeyman game might be played this way:

THE DOCTOR SAYS:
I'm afraid I can't help you.

THE BOGEYMAN WHISPERS:
He's telling you you're a hopeless case!

THE DOCTOR MEANT:
I'm a surgeon — and you don't need surgery.

THE PATIENT NEEDED TO HEAR:
You don't need surgery. I understand your condition is very painful and something must be done, but the solution is good back care and exercise, not an operation.

Some surgeons have the unfortunate habit of disowning patients who don't need surgery — which, in the case of back patients, is the vast majority. One surgeon I know likes to tell his patients, "I'm a cutting doctor, not a talking doctor." To me, that seems like the ultimate rejection of doctor-patient communication. But at least that surgeon leaves patients knowing where they stand. In contrast, the doctors who play Bogeyman arouse groundless fears that help perpetuate the false mystique of back pain.

Mum's the Word

This is a variation of Bogeyman. In this version of the game, the doctor simply leaves vital information unsaid by ignoring the patient's questions.

THE PATIENT ASKS:
Is there something seriously wrong with my spine?

THE DOCTOR (preoccupied with the x-rays) RESPONDS:
Did you ever have a fall?

THE BOGEYMAN WHISPERS:
He knows something! He's just groping for some way to break the bad news!

THE DOCTOR MEANT:
I don't think so, but it's too soon in the examination to be sure. The x-ray is interesting and I'd like a little more information.

THE PATIENT NEEDED TO HEAR:
There's no reason to think it's serious. Do you know that most people have back pain like this at some time in their lives?

Double Diagnosis

Two or more doctors can play. Each player takes a turn examining the same patient. All players must reach the same conclusion (diagnosis) but each must express it in entirely different terms. Object: maximum patient confusion. In its simplest form, Double Diagnosis is played this way:

PATIENT: What's wrong with my back, Dr. Smith?
DR. SMITH: You have facet arthritis.

SAME PATIENT (one month later): What's wrong with my back, Dr. Jones?
DR. JONES: You have spinal osteoarthrosis.

Dr. Smith and Dr. Jones are not disagreeing. Dr. Smith is saying that the patient has spinal joints that are inflamed. Dr. Jones is saying that there is something wrong with one or more of the patient's spinal joints. The only difference is that Dr. Jones's loftier phrase may cost the patient a few dollars more.

Even at that, this patient was relatively lucky, since only two doctors were playing. I knew a woman with a broken ankle who got into a game of Quadruple Diagnosis. She went to four doctors who all agreed on what was wrong. The trouble was, nobody told her they agreed. From Doctor One she learned that she had a spiral fracture. Doctor Two said it was an oblique break of the lower tibia. The third doctor called it a transverse crack with displacement. And the fourth labeled it a Pott's fracture.

There were no contradictions here. Spiral, oblique, and transverse merely describe the directions of various sections of the fracture. Pott was the first man to describe this type of fracture. The four doctors were simply stating the same problem in different terms, or seeing it from different points of view — a phenomenon that is not peculiar to medicine.

The confusion created by Double Diagnosis is compounded by certain patients. These are the pain-focused "doctor shoppers" who see physician after physician as they search for the "real" diagnosis and a physical source for their non-physical pain.

Crystal Ball

I know doctors who warn their patients, "Without an operation, you may wind up in a wheelchair or..." Then they go on to predict some dire consequence, such as a lifetime of pain or disability, or both.

A doctor who makes a prediction like that is playing the game I call Crystal Ball. In my view, it's risky and unfair. The risk to the doctor's credibility is obvious. We've all heard stories about people who have been told, "You'll never walk again," and who now, years later, are walking around as ably as ever and sneering at their doctors. Crystal Ball is especially risky with back patients because most bad backs get better without drastic treatment of any kind.

Why would a doctor utter such predictions? Usually, he's trying to coerce a patient to submit to a treatment he believes is right in the circumstances. But even if the prediction comes to pass, such tactics exert unfair pressure on the patient. Every mature patient has the right to hear a full and truthful description of any treatment and its risks and consequences before deciding whether to accept it. Perhaps your doctor has been making flat declarations about your future condition, suggesting that you will suffer unpleasant consequences unless you take this treatment or that. If so, my advice is to seek a second opinion. No good doctor will object.

I have also known doctors who play Crystal Ball not to talk a patient into an operation but to get rid of the patient. In this variation of the game, the doctor implies that an operation is really the only feasible remedy, but then he goes on to paint a lurid picture of how the operation could go wrong. This puts the patient in a bind — unwilling to risk the operation yet unable to get better without it. At this point, the patient usually looks for help elsewhere — which is just what the doctor wanted. But imagine the problem of persuading this patient to accept back surgery, should it really become necessary at some time in the future.

Thou Shalt Not

This game might also be called "Oh, You Helpless Cripple!" It's based on the premise that once you have back pain you might as well throw in the towel (but throw it very gently). No more fun for you. It's time to learn a list of "don'ts" as long as your arm — and remember: you ignore even one of them at your peril!

A back specialist I know hands his patients a list of Thou Shalt Nots that is so forbidding that it always reminds me of Alexander Woollcott's famous complaint that everything he liked was either illegal, immoral, or fattening. While the Bible manages with only Ten Commandments for all mankind, my colleague needs twice that number of Shalt Nots to control his back patients' behavior. And that's just his general list; there are supplementary strictures for vacuuming, sweeping, kitchen chores, laundry work, stair-climbing, and bed-making.

What's more, many of his rules are so impractical that they are laughable: "Don't reach." "Never lift anything weighing more than 15 pounds." "Don't get tired." How can anybody observe rules like these and still get on with the process of everyday living? Back patients need guidance, but in my opinion it's worse to have too many rules than to have no rules at all. A person faced with a ridiculous prohibition like "Don't reach" is unlikely to pay attention even to the reasonable rules on the list.

I was given a first-hand lesson in Thou Shalt Not long before I entered the medical profession. In my mid-teens I'd been having a little trouble with my sinuses, and so at my parents' urging I went to a doctor. He declared that the only way to clear up my condition was to avoid sweaty situations — no heavy physical exertion, no steamy showers, no humid locker-rooms. Now, I had just made the high-school football team, and here was a doctor telling me, in effect, Thou Shalt Not Behave Like a Football Player. Can you picture a young man following that advice just to clear up a bit of sinus trouble? Hardly. I simply ignored what he said and made sure my parents never found out. My sinuses, by the way, are fine.

Why do doctors dispense such unrealistic advice? Some, I think, naively believe that patients will give up comfortable habits and familiar pleasures just to feel better. And of course they won't, any more than I was willing to give up football. In other instances, especially with back cases, I think doctors issue Shalt Nots because they can't think of anything else to do. But, worst of all, I believe some doctors use rule making as a means of building an escape clause into their advice. After all, if a doctor's rules are numerous enough and stringent enough, some are sure to be broken sooner or later. Then, if the patient's pain recurs, guess who is left feeling guilty? Certainly not the doctor.

Santa Claus

What could be wrong with playing Santa Claus? When it comes to backache, there is plenty wrong with it. And it's a game that can be played all year round. Your doctor will try to give you everything you want to cure your back pain. You don't have to do anything; just lie back and someone else will take charge. The treatments are usually pleasant enough; pills to relax you or give you a nice buzz; massage or manipulation to work out those tight muscles; heat to reduce the painful tension, or traction to stretch out the spasm. Of course, the relief is only temporary and the pain will return, but that's all right because Santa will be there tomorrow to give you some more presents. After a while you become so dependent on the jolly old elf, you can't get rid of the pain any other way.

Creating dependency is a major concern in managing back pain. Like it or not, and most people don't, the only lasting solution to the problem is to take charge and deal with the pain yourself, on your own time. Sure you need help, but that should come in the form of supervision and advice, like a coach working with an athlete. Unless you have an active role and are prepared to take some responsibility, there can be no lasting improvement.

Then why would your doctor or physiotherapist or chiropractor play this game? Often it's a matter of control. It's good for the ego to have someone need you and when the practitioner begins to believe he possesses some innate skill or unique talent that the patient cannot duplicate, the game is on.

It's easy for patients to accept a passive role and it's easy for the doctors to give them one. How much more difficult is it to recommend the hard road of exercise and change in lifestyle? It takes more time, more persuasion, more effort, and it may not be successful. Given the choice, it's obvious why some doctors and patients will always play Santa Claus.

Ping-Pong

The most popular game on our list, Ping-Pong, will seem familiar to almost any reader who has been seeing back doctors for six months or more. Ping-Pong is described here in more detail than the other games because lengthy duration and endless variations in diagnosis and treatment are the very essence of the game. A good game of Ping-Pong can last for months, even years.

Any number of doctors and paramedics can play, and the more players there are, the more devastating the game. The object is to bat the patient back and forth as many times as possible before he realizes that he is the ping-pong ball.

In our play-by-play example below, the players are a family doctor (who gets an assist from a colleague on the opening serve), plus a physiotherapist, an orthopedic surgeon, and a psychiatrist. Their ping-pong ball is Charlie, forty-seven, a chartered accountant.

Readers who are aficionados of Ping-Pong are invited to take particular notice of the finesse of the orthopedic surgeon, who, at the first moment the ball is on his side of the net, manages to play, in rapid succession, five of the seven other games described earlier. Indeed, the opportunity to introduce one or more games-within-the-game strikes many players as one of Ping-Pong's most appealing features.

Notice, as well, that Ping-Pong employs a logbook rather than a scorecard. In the first few entries, I have inserted pings and pongs where they would likely occur. From Day 23 onward, I leave most of the sound effects to your imagination and note only the major tactical moves.

Day 1: Digging in his garden one Saturday, Charlie suffers a sudden attack of back pain. Unable to work, he watches TV and goes to bed early. The Ping-Pong game is about to begin.

Day 2: Charlie can hardly get out of bed. His back is killing him. He calls his family doctor but learns he is away for the weekend. The answering service refers him (ping) to Dr. White. With a supple forehand stroke, White scribbles a prescription. The pills, intended to work as pain-killers, only make Charlie sick to his stomach.

Day 3: Charlie sees his family physician, Dr. Brown. With a nonchalant backhand return, Brown writes a different prescription (pong); same medicine, different name, but these pills don't make Charlie sick.

Day 18: Even with sporadic relief provided by the pills, the pain drives Charlie back to Dr. Brown (ping). Brown deftly lobs him over to a physiotherapist (pong).

Day 23: The physiotherapist, Ms. Green, applies a hot pack and performs a massage (Santa Claus).

Days 23 to 37: In these two weeks, Charlie ricochets six times between his home and Ms. Green's office. The treatments feel good at the time but as he drives home, the car seat makes his back as painful as ever.

Day 38: Admitting failure with the hot packs and the massage (net serve), Ms. Green persuades Charlie to try ultrasound (defensive rally) to project heat painlessly into his spine.

Days 38 to 52: After each of his four trips in for ultrasound, his drive home is still murder on Charlie's back.

Day 55: Charlie returns to Dr. Brown's office (change of serve). Disturbed by Charlie's persistent pain, Brown bats him down the hall to X-Ray.

Day 56: Brown is puzzled: Charlie's x-rays are normal, yet his back still hurts. How can that be? He calls Charlie in (feint), recommends further examination (quick save), and flicks him over to an orthopedic surgeon.

Day 121: It's seventeen weeks since the game began. Having waited two months to see the orthopedic surgeon, Dr. Gray, Charlie receives a quick examination and a quicker verdict. Here, Gray deftly initiates five other games-within-the-game, beginning with a learned pronouncement: "You have unilateral spondylolysis" (Speaking Doctor). "I'm afraid there's nothing I can do for you" (Bogeyman). Ignoring Charlie's questions (Mum's the Word), Gray forehands him a three-page list of don'ts (Thou Shalt Not), and describes what will happen if he disregards them (Crystal Ball). (Gray does not play Double Diagnosis only because Charlie's condition has remained undiagnosed until now.) "You'll just have to live with your pain," Gray tells Charlie. He suggests checking back with Dr. Brown in a couple of weeks.

Day 133: It's Dr. Brown's serve, but he can't think of a new strategy. Forgetting momentarily what treatments Charlie has had, he suggests pills, hot packs, massage, ultrasound. . . . For the first time, Charlie distinctly hears the sound of the game in progress: ping-pong, ping-pong. He flares up but stops short. They're keeping something from him! He visualizes himself in a wheelchair. Bewildered and angry, he storms out of Dr. Brown's office.

Day 134: Charlie calls Dr. Brown, apologizes, and asks for more pills. He didn't sleep a wink all night. Brown gently suggests that the problem may be nerves. Unsure by now of his own mental stability, Charlie hasn't the stamina to argue when Brown refers him to a psychiatrist (forehand smash).

Day 168 to 318: In five months of weekly sessions with Dr. Black, Charlie probes his psyche back to early childhood. From this insight, Black makes a significant pronouncement: "There's nothing wrong with your head. You have back trouble. What you need is an orthopedic surgeon or at least a careful examination by your family doctor. When you get your back fixed up, you may want some psychotherapy. Come and see me then."

From here on, Charlie hears without heeding as the game's final rallies become a blur.

Day 332: Gray sees Charlie again and declares him unchanged: "As I said before, there's nothing I can do." (ping)

Day 339: Brown has heard of a new drug in Minnesota: "Unfortunately, the side effects . . ." (pong)

Day 353: Gray, just back from an international medical symposium, is high on a new surgical technique: "No guarantee, of course, but what else can we do? And what have you got to lose?" (ping)

Day 364: Brown recalls a spa in Arizona: "Pretty expensive, of course, but I've known patients who . . ." (pong)

Day 366: On the first anniversary of his back attack, Charlie riffles through the Yellow Pages and finds the listing he's looking for — Chiropractors. Then another thought strikes him: Frank, down at the office, was telling about this acupuncturist who . . .

Charlie's first Ping-Pong game is over. But he will soon get another one started — on his own.

The tragedy is that the treatment Charlie needs is simple, inexpensive, and undramatic. Given the right information, even yet, he could become his own most effective back doctor. All that's wrong with his back is a bit of wear from forty-seven years of living. The pain is real and the psychiatrist is right: there is nothing wrong with Charlie's head unless you count the anxiety that arises from back pain — and from Ping-Pong.

The treatments Charlie got — the pills, the hot packs, the massage, the ultrasound — were not necessarily useless, but they provided short-term relief at best. As for the long-term measures — the new surgical technique, the spa, the chiropractic, the acupuncture, even the wonder drug — any or all of them might have proved helpful, but Charlie could have done without them if he had been told, back on Day 3, what he really needed.

He needed a clear idea of what was wrong with his back — plus the assurance that his condition wasn't unusual or serious.

He needed frequent rest periods in positions that could rapidly reduce his pain.

He needed to learn a few simple, painless exercises that could be completed in a few minutes each day.

He needed a new set of daily habits — ways of sitting, standing, lifting, sleeping — to minimize the strain on his back.

He needed to realize that you don't cure a bad back — you control it.

It sounds far too simple and undramatic to be true. But it is true, as thousands of people have discovered for themselves.

Well, I can hear you saying, there has to be a catch to this somewhere. And you're right — there is a catch. While these simple steps could do wonders for Charlie and for most other people with back trouble, they're impossible to follow unless you understand what your back trouble is all about.

Now that we've dispelled the commonest myths and seen through Bogeyman and Ping-Pong and those other diversions that can sidetrack your efforts to find effective treatment, you're all set to start learning the things you need to know.

3 A Painless Course in Anatomy

I have already rejected the idea that your back is a mysterious and baffling part of your body. We know a great deal about the spine, and the more we learn, the more we appreciate what a truly marvelous piece of machinery it is.

That point was made in an amusing script written as part of a patient education video series for the Canadian Back Institute. The script is based upon a fanciful premise: a team of engineers is called upon to design a human back without ever having seen one. All that the engineers know at the outset is that some sort of scaffold is needed to support the human body. What could be simpler? They create a solid vertical model resembling a flagpole.

"Sorry," says the client, "but that won't do. Your spine has to be a lot more flexible than that."

The engineers scrap the pole design and fashion a stack of block-like bones. The bones articulate nicely but are forever slipping out of place. The designers hit on the idea of lashing them together with ligaments, the way thongs are lashed around the poles of wigwams.

"Wait a minute," says the client. "I forgot to tell you — the spine has to bend and rotate, like a construction crane." The engineers spend weeks adding pulleys and guy wires and designing an intricate system of interlocking joints. Several innovations are necessary, including a built-in lubrication system to prevent binding and squeaking, and a series of catches to prevent self-destruction through excessive rotation.

Each time they think they've created the perfect design, some new specification is added. The device has to bear considerable weight, not just at the top but down the sides, too. Their first answer to that challenge, a huge and ugly counterweight, is rejected out of hand. They add extra ligaments and muscles instead. The device has to withstand frequent jostling and bouncing up and down. They design discs as shock absorbers between the bones. It has to contain a built-in intercom system. They bore a hole down the center and install wires.

Their creation must have a lifting capacity of 300 pounds per square inch (21 kg per cm^2), yet the whole body, spine and all, should weigh no more than 150 pounds (68 kg) on the average, with some models at less than 100 pounds (45 kg). Quietly, they scrap their 8,000-pound (3600 kg) prototype without even unveiling it.

When they're told to make the whole thing mobile, they mount it on casters, but it keeps skidding about and tipping over. They haven't even solved that problem when the client begins talking wistfully of having "at least one model that can run a four-minute mile." At that point, they throw up their hands and resign en masse. Clearly, no device on earth could possibly meet all those specifications.

Once you consider the demands we place on our spines in the normal course of ordinary living, you no longer wonder why so many people have trouble with their backs. You wonder instead why everybody in the world doesn't suffer back pain.

Patients are always asking, "Why me? Why do I have to be the one with back trouble? Why can't I be normal?"

And I always tell them: "You are normal. It's normal to have back problems. The abnormal people are the ones who don't have back pain."

I always hasten to add that this is no reason to put up with a bad back. But the first part is true: anybody who lives an average lifespan without suffering from backache belongs to a privileged minority. By projecting the statistics on back problems, I have calculated that on any given day, about eleven million people in the United States and Canada are suffering from backache.

Why are so many people susceptible? The answer
begins to emerge when you see how your spine is put
together, what strains are imposed on it, and what
changes it undergoes as your body ages. Marvelous
though it is, your spine has its potential weak spots, and
if you want to protect them from abuse and prevent them
from causing pain, it's important to know where these
weaknesses are and how they develop.

As we all know, your spine consists basically of bones
called vertebrae, which are separated and cushioned by
oval pads called discs. From the base of your skull through
to the bottom of your tailbone, you have thirty-three or
thirty-four vertebrae contained in five sections or regions.
The three upper regions, which form the mobile part of
your spine, have twenty-four vertebrae among them. The
two lower regions have nine or ten bones in two fused sections. You have seven vertebrae in your neck or cervical
region; twelve in the mid-back, known as the thoracic or
dorsal region (these are the vertebrae attached to your
ribs), and five vertebrae, the largest of the lot, in the low
back or lumbar region. The two immobile sections are the
sacrum and the coccyx. (The latter term, pronounced
"cock-six," is Latin for cuckoo; the coccyx resembles a
cuckoo's bill.) During the formative months before birth,
your sacrum was five individual bones, but by the time
you were born, it had fused into a single bone. Since the
sacrum forms the back of your pelvis, it does not require
the flexibility of the spinal regions above it. Finally, you
have four or five bones in your tailbone or coccyx. Many
people are intrigued to learn that some of us have four
coccyx bones while others have five. The coccyx is all
that's left of the tail we inherited from the apes a few million years ago, and if you happen to have five coccyx
bones, you can perhaps consider yourself a closer relation
to our ancient forebears than people who have only four.

I seldom rhyme off the names of these spinal regions to
an audience without telling a favorite story of mine. It
involves a new medical secretary who had a little trouble
deciphering her notes from a dictated letter, specifically a

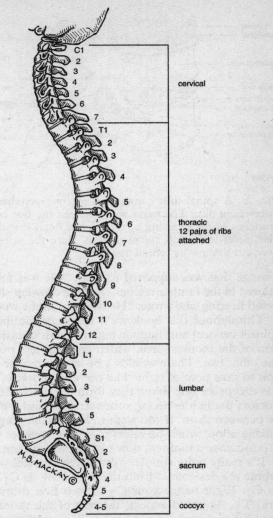

Fig. 1. A side view of the full spine and the five named regions. The cervical and lumbar regions are the most flexible and are the sites of most back pain.

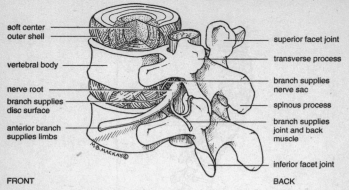

soft center
outer shell

superior facet joint

vertebral body

transverse process

branch supplies
nerve sac

nerve root

branch supplies
disc surface

spinous process

anterior branch
supplies limbs

branch supplies
joint and back
muscle

inferior facet joint

M.B.MACKAY©

FRONT   BACK

Fig. 2. A spinal unit consists of any two vertebrae and the intervening disc. The nerve root between the two bones sends branches to the covering of the nerves, outer one-third of the disc, facet joint, and spinal muscle. Here the upper disc has been cut to show its central nucleus.

passage that was supposed to read, "He was found to be injured in the lumbar region." Relying on what she remembered hearing, she wrote: "He was shot in the woods."

Throughout this book we'll be concentrating on your spine's cervical and lumbar regions, with occasional mention of the thoracic area, which gives far less trouble than the other two. There wouldn't be any particular reason for you to take note of terms like cervical, thoracic, and lumbar except for one thing: they form the basis of the system doctors use in identifying your vertebrae and the discs that lie between them. If you want to know what your doctor is talking about when he refers to a T_{12} vertebra or an L_2-L_3 disc, take a moment now to learn this system.

It's really quite simple. Your seven cervical (neck) vertebrae are designated from the top down, as C_1, C_2, etc., to C_7. Right below your C_7 is your first thoracic vertebra, T_1. As you'd expect, the rest of the thoracic vertebrae are numbered downward to T_{12}, and then the lumbars take over: L_1 to L_5.

Each disc and the adjacent pair of joints derive their designation from the vertebrae above and below them. Hence

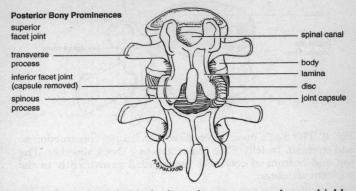

Posterior Bony Prominences

superior
facet joint

transverse
process

inferior facet joint
(capsule removed)

spinous
process

spinal canal

body

lamina

disc

joint capsule

M B MACKAY ©

Fig. 3. Seen from behind, the spine presents a bony shield, which protects the contents of the spinal canal. The tough capsule enclosing each facet joint adds extra stability. The bony projections to each side are for muscle attachment.

the disc lying between your third and fourth lumbar vertebrae is called your L_3-L_4 disc. This designation is often abbreviated further as simply L_3-$_4$. Similarly, the disc between your lowest thoracic vertebra and your uppermost lumbar vertebra is called the T_{12}-L_1 disc accompanied by the T_{12}-L_1 joints. The lowest disc in your spine is the L_5-S_1 — that is, the disc between the lowest of the five lumbar vertebrae and the first of the fused sacral segments. Although the sacrum shows signs of having originated as five separate bones, it contains no discs.

That's all there is to it. And if you feel that your doctor is "Speaking Doctor" unnecessarily when he uses these designations, remember that though it may sound technical and mysterious, it's the only brief and accurate way of identifying your spinal bones, discs, and nerves. Otherwise, instead of saying, "Your pain originates at your L_4 level," your doctor would have to say, "at the twenty-third vertebra from the top," or "the fourth vertebra of your lumbar region."

Now let's take a look at your spine and identify the potential trouble spots.

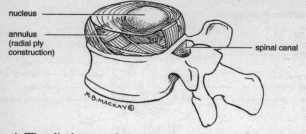

Fig. 4. The disc's outer layers have a radial ply construction to add strength. Its jelly-filled center acts as a shock absorber. The top and bottom of each disc are bonded permanently to the adjacent vertebrae.

Each vertebra looks like a squat little drum with an upright tube fastened to its back. The drum sits with its flat surfaces at the top and bottom. Extending from the walls of the tube are several odd-looking projections. Three of these projections are spike-shaped bones — two extending sideways like wings, and the third, with a knobby end on it, pointing straight back. This third spike, and others like it on the other vertebrae, are the knobby bones that can be felt when you run your fingers up and down your back or somebody else's. This is the only part of the backbone you can feel from outside your body. And while those knobby ends may feel as though they are just under the skin, they are actually well below the surface — about half an inch (1 cm) below in a thin person and as much as 2 inches (5 cm) below in an overweight one. Which means it's a long way in from the surface of your skin to the center of the drum-shaped part of your vertebra and to the center of the adjacent disc — perhaps 3 inches (7.5 cm) in a person of normal weight and maybe 5 or 6 inches (13 or 15 cm) in a heavy person. That's a critical point to keep in mind whenever someone talks as though the spine were something just under the skin to grab hold of and move around.

Between the drum-shaped sections of the vertebrae lie the discs. Each disc is tightly bonded, top and bottom, to the adjacent vertebrae above and below — so tightly that it cannot possibly slip out of place the way some people imagine. This bonding effect is so strong, in fact, that if you suffered an extreme blow to your spine — say, in an automobile accident — the vertebral bones would likely give way before any of the discs would fail. By separating and cushioning the vertebrae from each other, the disc helps support the weight of your head and upper body and absorbs the shock of any unusual load or sudden downward pressure.

If you could examine a disc, you would find that it has a tough elastic shell made of criss-crossed layers of fibers like the plies in a radial tire. In fact, you might even wonder whether the designers of modern automobile tires got the idea from studying spinal discs. If you looked inside the disc, you would find a soft substance about the consistency of jelly. And, like the jelly desserts you make from powders, this material is mostly water.

Water trapped in the center of the disc (an area called the nucleus) is slowly but constantly exchanged. Chemical attraction draws fluid from the surrounding tissue and the force of gravity pushes it back out. This ebb and flow carries necessary nutrients into the disc and removes waste products. The process is assisted by body movement. The more you move your back, the more you feed your discs.

Since it's the water that gives the disc its cushiony character, much like the water in a waterbed, you can imagine what happens if the disc dries up. The loss of the hydraulic shock-absorber effect is a major source of back pain.

Each vertebra has two pairs of bony parts jutting towards the back of your body. One pair extends from the top corners of the tube, the other pair from the bottom corners. The lower projections extend downward to interlock with the upper projections of the vertebra below. Where these projections make contact, they form the joints called facet joints. In that manner, each vertebra is interlocked with its neighbors, in two long, parallel ridges of interlocking joints on either side of the ridge of your back bone. Between these interlocking joints, the outer wall of each vertebral tube — that is, the part of the wall closest to the skin of your back — overlaps its neighbor below, like the overlapping scales of a fish. These overlapping walls (called laminae) along with the interlocking joints and the bony projections described earlier, form a shield of bone that protects the contents of the spinal canal.

The projections that form the facet joints are capped with cartilage — the same kind of smooth white cartilage you have seen on the knobby end of a chicken leg. The cartilage is incredibly smooth, hundreds of times smoother than the moving parts in a high-performance engine. And it is self-lubricating. Movement and pressure force a slick, oily substance in and out of the joint surface. The joints are maintained and nourished by movement. The purpose of the cartilage, of course, is to permit easy, almost friction-free movement of the joints, which are about the size of the joints in your fingers. Each joint is tightly encased in a strong, fibrous capsule that prevents the joint from coming part. The joint is so secure inside its capsule that it is easier to dislocate your shoulder than to dislocate a facet joint.

All in all, it's a highly effective joint system. If the smooth surfaces of the joints become roughened through wear, however, or if a joint tightens up under pressure, the bones grind against each other, and you've got joint pain.

Let's take a closer look at the tube-like structure on the back of the drum — the part known as the spinal canal, which encases your spinal cord. Most people think of the canal as a cylinder-like pipeline. In reality, it is a five-sided tunnel resembling the outline of one of those little houses used in playing Monopoly. The sloping sides that look like the roof of the house are the laminae, which help form that protective shield we described earlier. Figure 5 shows this shape clearly. Notice how closely the "floor" of the house is positioned to the drum-shaped part of the vertebra and to the adjacent disc. As long as that disc retains its shape, the system functions well; if it doesn't, you're looking at another trouble spot.

As you might expect, your back muscles also play a part in any back problem you may have. But, contrary to what you may have always assumed, your spine does not have one long muscle running from top to tailbone. Most of your back muscles are fairly small, working in pairs or threesomes, each spanning only two or three vertebrae. The only really large muscle in your back is the one that weight-lifters work so hard to develop. It's called the trapezius, and it's a kite-shaped structure, with one point at the tip of your skull, two opposite points at the outer edges of your shoulders, and the fourth point halfway down the center of your back.

Your back muscles can be associated with back pain in three ways, all of them involving spasm, a tensing-up commonly referred to as a muscle cramp. The muscular spasms that occur in your back are essentially the same as those familiar, painful cramps we all get at times in our calves through to the arches of our feet. In your back, a spasm may occur as a muscular reaction to a small tear in the outer shell of a disc. Or, even without a physical cause, a back muscle may go into spasm in response to emotional stress. Or, a muscle already in spasm may cause other muscles to go into spasm, thereby radiating tension and pain to other parts of your spine.

And of course there is a close relationship between back pain and the nerves in and around your spine. In some instances, a nerve itself may be the actual site of your trouble, if it is being irritated by pressure from some other part of the spine, such as a disc. More commonly, a nerve, or several nerves, may simply be serving as the "telephone lines" communicating the message from the nerve ends to the brain, signaling that such-and-such a body part is being pressed, squeezed, rubbed, or otherwise irritated. So let's take a look at your nervous system and see in more detail how it relates to your back problems.

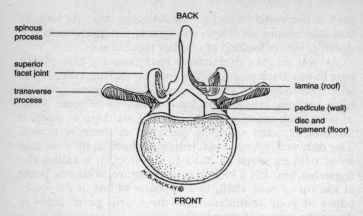

spinous
process

superior
facet joint

transverse
process

BACK

lamina (roof)

pedicule (wall)

disc and
ligament (floor)

M.S. MACKAY©

FRONT

Fig. 5. The five-sided shape of the spinal canal resembles a
Monopoly house. The floor of the canal is alternately bone on
the back of the vertebra and a strong ligament covering the
intervertebral disc. Two facet joints and three bony prominences project from the roof; these are for muscle attachment.

If you've ever peeked inside an old-style television set
and seen the confusing array of wire "spaghetti" that pre-
dated printed circuitry, you can begin to imagine the
great complexity of nerves centered in your spinal cord.

All along your spinal canal there are small openings
between the bony projections of adjacent vertebrae.
These openings serve as passages for pairs of nerves
branching out, right and left, from the spinal cord. These
main branches, or nerve roots as they are often called,
split off into lesser branches, some to serve the spine
itself, others the limbs and the rest of the body.

The spinal cord is an extension of your brain that
protrudes through a hole in the base of your skull and
runs down inside the spinal canal. It is slightly smaller
than your little finger and is wrapped in several thin
membranes. The spinal cord ends at the upper end of
the lumbar region, just below your ribs. From there
down to the pelvis, the canal is filled only with nerve
roots, which have left the cord but have not yet left the

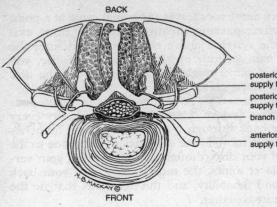

BACK

posterior branch
supply to muscle

posterior branch
supply to facet joint

branch supply to disc

anterior branch
supply to trunk and limbs

M.B.MACKAY ©

FRONT

Fig. 6. Branches of the spinal nerve roots supply the dural sac around the nerves, the outer layers of the disc, the facet joints, and the back muscle. As it leaves the spinal canal to supply a limb, each nerve root must pass directly over the back corner of the disc.

spine. To the early anatomists, this tangle of nerves looked like the tail of a horse, hence its name, cauda equina, or horse's tail.

The nerves of your spine are divided into the same sections as the vertebrae and are given the same designations — C_1, T_1, L_1, and so on — but with one minor variation. Because there are eight cervical nerves, compared with only seven cervical vertebrae, the C series for the nerves runs to C_8, while the C series for the vertebrae stops at C_7.

Nerve roots from the lower cervical area come together to form major branches that pass below your shoulders and into your arms. For this reason, if you have trouble in your neck, you may feel pain in your shoulder. Similarly, nerve roots exiting from the lower lumbar and upper sacral areas join together to form the sciatic nerve, which runs down the back of your leg. This explains why you sometimes suffer leg pains as a result of trouble in your lower back.

Since every nerve root leaves the spinal canal at a point close to a disc, passing through a narrow bony exit formed by the vertebra above and below, and since the size of that exit depends on the height of the disc, you can see how a nerve might get into trouble if the disc bulges in the wrong place.

Apart from its service to the rest of your body, your central nervous system is connected to virtually every part of your back through a network of small branches from each nerve root. These connections are made to the outer part of your disc (though not the center), your vertebrae and facet joints, the muscles that give your back movement and flexibility, and the ligaments that tie the whole structure together.

Although most people think of the spinal cord as merely a conduit between the brain and the body, it in fact carries out certain functions that were once credited exclusively to the brain. When your doctor gives you that familiar reflex test by tapping your knee lightly with a rubber mallet, the impulses race up your nerves as far as the spinal cord — but no farther. Your spinal cord responds to the impulse by "ordering" a muscular reaction.

In response to back pain, your spinal cord performs an intermediate function, processing raw information received from the nerve ends, and relaying this information, in more refined form, to the brain.

It's a system that could be compared to the creation of a simple photograph. At the scene of the picture-taking, light enters the lens to record an image on the film. Carried into the darkroom, the film is processed by a technician who neither knows nor cares what it depicts. Finally the picture is passed along to the photographer, who is the first to identify the likeness of lovable old Aunt Tilly squinting at us from her front porch. With back pain, the sequence is: impulses at the nerve ends, processing in the spinal cord — in the dark, so to speak — and identification of the message by the brain as pain.

Every communications system has its limitations, and in this one, the spinal cord can't tell which of the mini-branches and secondary branches carried that message into the main nerve branch. This is one reason why a doctor may find it difficult to localize a back problem from what you can say about where you feel your pain. You may have to admit, "I don't know whether the pain is coming from my calf, from behind my knee or from the back of my thigh." When that happens, you are experiencing the phenomenon doctors call referred pain.

There are other reasons why you may be misled about the source of your pain. For instance, that big trapezius muscle on your upper back may pick up pain sensations from your lower back and transmit them to the back of your neck. Or your back muscles may create additional pain in a secondary area by reacting to irritation felt by, say, a facet joint. When the joint irritation is translated into pain by the spinal cord, the muscles at the scene of the trouble may respond by tightening up. This is a protective reaction intended to immobilize the irritated area and thus prevent further irritation. Ironically, however, this reaction may be so severe that it produces pain of its own. You may not recognize this condition for what it is — a muscle spasm or cramp; you may think your whole back has "gone out." And unless you know more than most people know about back problems, you probably wouldn't believe me if I told you that the culprit in this whole affair is just one tiny, but irritable, spinal joint no bigger than the joint in one of your thumbs.

Here's how a little case of facet joint pain in the lumbar area can be magnified:

1. The pain, caused by normal wear, originates in a small joint.

2. The initial impulse is transmitted into the main nerve and along to the spinal cord, where it is processed as back pain.

3. The impulse courses throughout the length of the nerve, which, as it happens, also runs down into the leg. Now you have leg pain as well as back pain.

4. The muscles in the affected area react by going into spasm. Now you have muscular pain as well as leg pain and back pain.

5. Because the action is taking place on one side of your body, your spine is forced to curve unnaturally to that side as the muscles contract.

6. Other muscles respond by tightening up in new spasms. You are now virtually immobile.

In short, one little trouble spot in the facet joint becomes responsible for creating back pain, leg pain, muscular pain in various locations, and loss of movement of one side, and possibly both sides, of your body. No wonder your doctor may have trouble diagnosing your problem, and no wonder you're convinced that you have something far more serious than simple irritation of a spinal joint. And isn't it easy to see why so many people are frightened unnecessarily by a condition that can be traced to a source that is not permanent and that, in itself, is not even serious?

You may be wondering whether the things I've been saying about low back pain apply as well to neck pain. In general, the answer is yes. There are differences, however, that have to do with mobility and your awareness of what's going on in that portion of your spine.

Your neck, being designed for greater mobility than the lower parts of your spine, is obviously more susceptible to any trouble arising from movement between the vertebrae. And since the cervical or neck region of your spine is closer to the surface and encased in less fat and muscles, you are always more aware of anything that is going on there. Even here, of course, your spine is a good distance under the skin. It usually comes as a surprise to learn that the distance from the back of the neck to the center of the disc is about the same as the distance from the disc center to the front of the neck. Still, your neck may readily emit the cracking sounds that occur harmlessly with the normal movement of your spinal joints, and you will hear those sounds more easily because the joints are covered with a thinner layer of tis-

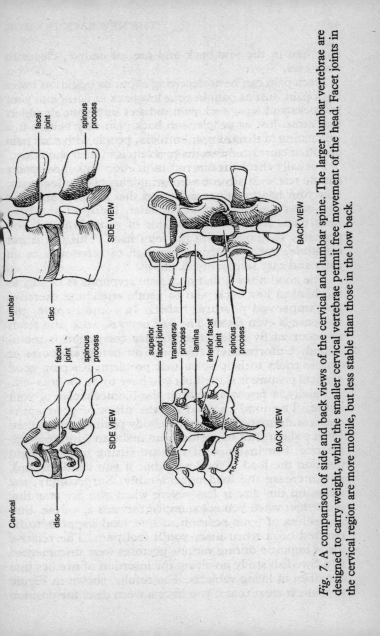

Cervical

facet
joint

spinous
process

disc

SIDE VIEW

disc

SIDE VIEW

Lumbar

facet
joint

spinous
process

superior
facet joint

transverse
process

lamina

inferior facet
joint

spinous
process

BACK VIEW

BACK VIEW

M.B.MAKAR©

Fig. 7. A comparison of side and back views of the cervical and lumbar spine. The larger lumbar vertebrae are designed to carry weight, while the smaller cervical vertebrae permit free movement of the head. Facet joints in the cervical region are more mobile, but less stable than those in the low back.

sue than in the low back and are, of course, closer to your ears.

Neck pain can be as deceiving about its origins as lower back pain. Just as pain in your low back radiates into your buttocks and legs, neck pain radiates into your shoulders and arms. Just as people with back pain may believe it is originating in their hips or buttocks, people with neck pain are often convinced that the problem is in their shoulders.

I usually check for this radiation effect by conducting a simple test with anyone who complains of shoulder pain: take your hand and cover the part that is most painful. If you cover the top of your shoulder, I suspect you have neck pain. If you cover the side of your shoulder, you probably have pain from the joint itself. This test is not infallible, but it's accurate enough to serve well as an early and easy step in my diagnosis.

The good news is that neck pain responds as rapidly as mechanical low back pain to gentle stretching exercises and improved postural habits. In some people, the response is even faster. The bad news is, neck pain tends to recur easily unless the posture correction is maintained. Unfortunately there are no handy supports or simple tricks to help solve that problem. Keeping good cervical posture is something you have to do for yourself.

Finally, a few words about the biomechanics of your spine. The load exerted on the discs of your spine changes dramatically from one body position to another. Even a slight shift in position can make an enormous difference. For instance, if you are sitting in an upright position the load is moderate, but if you bend forward, you increase the load considerably. Surprisingly, the stress on the disc is less severe when you are standing erect than when you are slumped forward at a desk. But, regardless of your position, if that load happens to be exerted on a worn disc, you'll feel pain. The relative loads imposed during various postures were documented in a Swedish study involving the insertion of needles into the discs of living subjects. The results, shown in Figure 8, make it clear that if you have a worn disc, the position

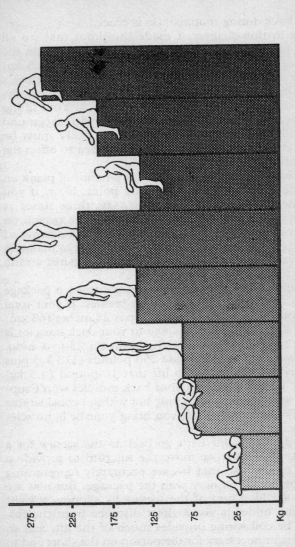

Fig. 8. This diagram illustrates the relative pressures within the third lumbar disc in various positions. Pressure is least while lying on the back and greatest while sitting forward. Interdiscal pressure is generally higher when sitting than when standing. (After Nachemson)

of your back during routine tasks is crucial.

Early in this chapter, I made the point that we all impose incredible demands upon our backs, just in the course of everyday living. Imagine a 10-pound (4.5 kg) package sitting on a table. You reach out to lift it at arm's length. In holding your arm out, away from your body, you automatically use muscles in your back. Your lifting action becomes comparable to the action of a playground seesaw. If the package is to be raised, there must be enough downward thrust in your spinal area to offset the weight of the package and provide lift.

Ordinarily, a seesaw has the same amount of plank on each side of the fulcrum, or center point. Now, if you move the fulcrum so that there is, say, three times as much plank on one side as on the other, the person on the short end has to exert three times as much downward pressure (or add that much extra weight) just to maintain equilibrium. In other words, he's working against a ratio of three to one.

The same principle applies when you raise a package at arm's length, but the ratio is far greater. If your total reach from mid-spine to finger grasp is 25 inches (63 cm) and the distance from mid-spine to your back muscles is 1 inch (2.5 cm), you're working against a 25-to-1 ratio. That means you must provide 250 pounds (113 kg) plus of downward thrust just to lift that 10-pound (4.5 kg) package. Chances are that your back muscles won't supply that much force — certainly not without considerable strain. To spread the load, you bring your belly muscles into play.

How do they help? Let's go back to the seesaw for a moment. This time we move the fulcrum to provide a 25-to-1 ratio — so that we are accurately representing the lift problem you have with the package. But now we support the long arm of the seesaw by slipping a giant coil spring under it just a short distance from the fulcrum. The coil spring provides much of the lift, and so it's no longer necessary for the person on the short end to exert the entire 250-pound (113 kg) downward pressure.

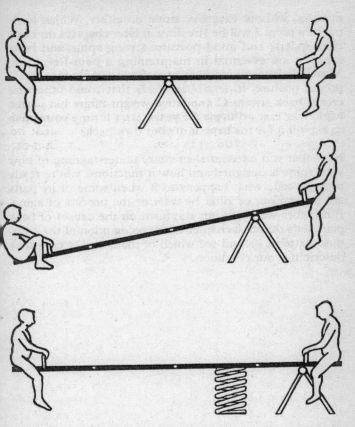

Fig. 9. With the same length on each side, the seesaw is balanced by two people of the same weight. As the lengths change, the balance is lost. Additional support from the spring helps solve the problem without increasing the load on the short side.

Your belly muscles can perform much the same function as that coil spring. By tightening those muscles during the lift, you redistribute some of the exertion, so that the load is shared by your back muscles and your belly muscles, without excessive strain on either. Which leads me to a point I will be stressing in later chapters on exercise, sports, and good posture: strong spine and belly muscles are essential in maintaining a pain-free back. Muscle balance around your trunk not only helps sustain proper posture, it distributes loads that could otherwise create back strain. Competitive weight-lifters have been exploiting that principle for years. Isn't it time you began to exploit it for the benefit of your own back?

Now that you have an elementary understanding of how your spine is designed and how it functions, you're ready to appreciate what happens to it when some of its parts are thrown out of kilter by wear or the process of aging. But before we begin our rundown on the causes of back pain, let's devote a chapter to the recognition of the common patterns — and see which of them comes closest to describing your condition.

4 Are You Pattern One, Two, Three, or Four?

Suppose that you and I had never met until you walked up to me at a social gathering and said, "Hello, I'm so-and-so. I understand that you're a back specialist. I have this pain right here in my lower back. What do you think is wrong?"

Now, in the best medical tradition — and to cut down on my malpractice costs — I'd feel obliged to reply, "I'm sorry, but I wouldn't hazard a guess without first discussing your medical history and symptoms and examining you in my office."

Secretly I'd be tempted to say, "I'll bet you nine to one that you've got either a painful disc or a worn facet joint."

How can I be so sure? Well, I wouldn't really know. But my informed guess would be a pretty safe bet. First, I would assume that you hadn't injured your back in a recent significant accident; if you had, you wouldn't be asking me what was wrong — you'd already know. Second, I'd assume that your back problem was not part of a generalized disease. If it were, you might have other symptoms and you wouldn't likely describe your condition simply as back pain.

By deduction and knowing the odds, I would conclude that you probably have one of the two common patterns of back-dominant pain, conditions I call Pattern One and Pattern Two. The current evidence suggests that these two mechanical patterns are related to problems in the discs or small joints. Together they account for about ninety percent of the back-pain stories that I hear. Incidentally, the term "mechanical" in this context means pain arising from the structural elements of the spine, not from an infection, disease, or tumor. It is pain clearly altered by movement and position. The other common patterns, Pattern Three and Pattern Four, produce leg-dominant pain, where the leg pain is worse than the pain in the back. Taken together, the latter two patterns account for only ten percent of cases. And remember, you did say "back pain."

So you can see that while my silent and instant diagnosis of your trouble wasn't foolproof — deduction seldom is — statistically, I had a very good chance of being right. An experienced doctor makes judgments of this sort every day. He begins a diagnosis with the broad assumption that a patient's condition is as commonplace as the obvious symptoms suggest. As he proceeds with the diagnosis, he protects himself and his patient from the danger of error by including observations and tests that will either rule out or point to some less common condition. And of course if there is evidence of an unusual problem, he'll take special steps to check on it. Since his days in medical school, however, he has had it drummed into his head that "common things happen most commonly." And he has probably heard the same principle enunciated in the expression, "When you hear hoofbeats, think horses, not zebras."

Most of us follow that principle in the course of everyday living, whether we realize it or not. Suppose, for instance, that you have a house guest who is about to borrow your car. He walks out with your key and two minutes later comes back to say that the car won't start. Immediately, you assume that it's just some minor problem: maybe the car is out of gas, or the battery is low, or the carburetor is acting up. You don't jump to the conclusion that the engine block is cracked or that the pistons have suddenly seized up. These things happen to automobiles, but you don't assume at the outset that your car has serious trouble.

We all apply that sort of common sense when we have trouble with our cars. But, for some reason, when people have trouble with their backs, common sense flies out the window. Instead of assuming that their trouble is ordinary, minor, and temporary, people allow the pain to convince them that they must have some dread disease.

If you have been harboring that sort of fear about your back condition, I urge you to reconsider: in the absence of any evidence to the contrary, try assuming for the time being that you have one of the common forms of back trouble. For what I am proposing to do here is to help you discover, by yourself, whether your problem is Pattern One, Pattern Two, Pattern Three, or Pattern Four.

You will have plenty of opportunity later to let your doctor explore the rarer possibilities, if he sees any reason to do so. In any case, there's no risk involved in checking your condition against the descriptions I give you here; in fact, the exercise will help prepare you to answer your own doctor's questions more accurately and precisely, thereby saving time and avoiding any misunderstanding that could hamper diagnosis and delay treatment.

It should almost go without saying that I don't expect you to conduct a self-examination while you are in severe pain. If you are immobilized with muscle spasms or emotionally upset by your pain, put this book aside and come back to it after you've rested enough to be on the road to temporary recovery. My questions and tests are intended for use while your pain is present but more or less tolerable, or while you are waiting patiently for your next acute attack.

Let's begin by making sure that your pain is originating in your back, not in your hip — which is one of the sites most often confused with back pain. Try these two tests.

Lying on your back, draw your knees up to your chest. If that causes pain in your groin, you may have hip trouble.

Now, with the knees still bent, turn your lower legs out. If that gentle twisting motion hurts, again you may have hip trouble. In that case, the twist of your leg will cause typical pain in your groin and perhaps down the front of your thigh to the knee. The hip rarely produces pain felt mainly in the buttock; the common patterns of back pain do.

No problem so far? Then let's move on to rule out trauma as the cause of your back pain. If you can't remember being injured, your back problem is not a case of accidental damage. Any accident serious enough to continue to cause severe pain weeks or months later would be a major and memorable incident: perhaps an auto collision, a substantial fall, or a serious incident such as the war injury that caused John F. Kennedy back pain for years.

With trauma eliminated, what about disease? You can probably rule that out too, if you can answer yes to all four of these questions:

1. Does your back feel better after a good rest?
2. Does each acute attack of pain pretty well disappear in about two weeks? (Recognizing that another attack could occur soon after the first one.)
3. Are you free of accompanying symptoms such as fever; weight loss; skin rashes; problems with other joints, particularly in your fingers, toes, hips, and knees; or persistent morning stiffness in your back even after the pain is gone?
4. Is your pain made worse by specific activities such as sitting or bending in one direction and does it diminish if you can find the right rest position? In other words, is your pain related to posture and activity?

Even if you answered no to one or two of those questions, your problem is not necessarily a disease. The odds remain strongly in favor of common backache.

If you have passed the test so far, you can be reasonably certain that you have Pattern One, Two, Three, or Four back pain or, at most, some combination of them. The first two patterns, by the way, are what our forefathers used to call lumbago, which is an archaic term meaning low back pain.

To help determine what pattern of backache you have, study the descriptions that follow. Be sure to read all four descriptions because their symptoms and characteristics overlap to some extent. In fact, during the acute phase it may be impossible to distinguish the pain of one pattern from that of another. Also, take note that although these descriptions are typical, they cannot apply to everyone's case of common back pain. Unusual variations may develop to create symptoms that are not typical. Besides, some people have more than one pattern and others experience varying symptoms over time because they are affected by two or more patterns in succession.

See which of these descriptions comes closest to defining your form of back pain.

Pattern One

Your trouble may begin with a lift or twist, or a minor incident of routine exertion, such as picking up a garden hose or retrieving a golf ball. You may recall no event at all. The pain often starts as a knot or pulling sensation in your back and increases slowly. By the end of the first day, your back is very sore; by the second day it's even worse. Your pain is felt mainly in the low back or buttocks, but it can, and often does, radiate into the legs. Your symptoms are increased by bending forward or sitting, and may be relieved by arching backward. Once established, the back pain can last for weeks or even months.

In a few cases, Pattern One can have a sudden onset and run the brief episodic course more typical of Pattern Two. But the aggravating effect of bending forward and the location of the dominant back pain remain the same.

If you were asked to place your hands on the most painful area, you would probably reach back to indicate the top of your buttocks. If you exert a little pressure there, you can easily feel two bony lumps located at the top of your pelvis. These lumps are normal, of course; they are at the upper points of your sacroiliac joints.

These are not the points where your pain is originating, but your muscle spasm makes it feel as though they were. Sacroiliac joints used to be blamed for a great deal of back pain a few years ago, before doctors learned more about sacroiliac function and the sources of Pattern One pain.

Pattern Two

Pattern Two has some similarity to Pattern One. Your dominant pain is again in the back or buttocks. Leg symptoms are common, but the pain there is a secondary complaint. The attack may be almost immediate or its intensity may increase rapidly. Your pain is accentuated when you arch your back, as you do when you lean back to look up at the ceiling. The pain increases as the movement is repeated. Your symptoms may reduce when you bend forward.

With rest, or at least in the absence of any aggravation, your acute pain disappears within four to fourteen days. This pattern of recovery is welcome, but it can also be embarrassing. Many a Pattern Two patient has been in great agony while arranging a doctor's appointment, only to find the pain gone on the day of the visit. Don't be embarrassed if this happens to you. Keep your appointment anyway and report the sequence of events. A good back doctor won't be surprised to hear that your pain has come and gone, and he will use the information as an important clue in your diagnosis.

Your attack may never recur. But if it does, its most typical pattern will be recurrences two or three times a year.

An uncommon variation of Pattern Two is more chronic in nature, developing slowly over several days and lasting for weeks or months, a picture more typical of Pattern One. However, the principal features of Pattern Two remain: pain felt most severely in the back and aggravated by repeatedly bending backward.

The One-Two Combination

So far, we have dealt with Patterns One and Two as separate entities, which in fact they are. The causes of these two types of backache, however, are closely interrelated, as you will discover in the next chapter. And because of this close relationship, it is possible for you to have a combination of Pattern One and Pattern Two. To test this possibility, check your history carefully.

Do you find you have acute, short-term attacks interspersed with longer-lasting attacks? Perhaps you have noticed that not all your attacks begin in the same way or last the same amount of time.

Is your pain aggravated when you bend forward and backward? Is straightening up from a forward bent position the most painful movement of all? If so, you could have two separate patterns of pain. Your problem is not necessarily any worse if you have both types in combination, but it can be more difficult to diagnose and more frustrating to treat.

A Negative Test for Patterns One and Two

Most readers will identify with the symptoms of either Pattern One or Pattern Two, since these account for nine out of every ten cases of common back pain. Readers who don't feel that their condition has been described so far may be tempted to skip ahead from here to see whether their symptoms are set out under Pattern Three or Pattern Four. Instead, I suggest that every reader take the simple test I describe next, because it provides a useful clue about all four patterns of pain.

This test will be negative in cases of Pattern One or Two back pain; that is, it will not cause pain if your problem is only Pattern One or Two. It is also negative in people with Pattern Four leg-dominant pain. Therefore, it can be used by someone with any of these problems to confirm that they do not have Pattern Three, the pinched nerve. Obviously, readers who believe they may have Pattern Three ought to try this test too.

Leg pain worse than back pain indicates symptoms coming from direct pressure on a nerve root. This is typically the case in Patterns Three and Four. It is important to understand that a nerve can be subjected to pressure without losing its ability to function. When we talk about these two patterns of back pain, we are referring to symptoms that merely indicate that a nerve is being irritated; the nerve's function may or may not have been disrupted. If nerve conduction has been impaired, you have a greater amount of pressure than is required to produce irritation alone. It is acute painful irritation of a nerve, however, that distinguishes Pattern Three from the other patterns of common backache. The following test, described in two parts, is designed specifically to determine whether you have an acutely irritated spinal nerve.

A. Lying on your back, try lifting one leg with the knee straight. If you cannot manage the lift alone, have someone help raise the leg gently for you. Does this action produce your typical leg pain? If you have Pattern Three, the pain caused by leg lifting will be felt in the back of your thigh, the back of your knee, or even down to your toes. This test may cause back pain, but that is not significant; it's the typical leg pain, or lack of it, that matters. All the back pain indicates is the presence of Pattern One or Pattern Two trouble in the back itself, which, no doubt, you already recognize.

B. Now take note of the degree to which you can lift that leg, or allow it to be lifted for you. Don't expect to lift it to form a right angle, which is ninety degrees; only people who do this exercise regularly can manage that. But can you manage to lift it more than two-thirds of a right angle, that is, more than sixty degrees, without leg pain? If so, you are likely to have Pattern One or Two rather than Pattern Three.

Pattern Three

People think of a pinched nerve as a condition entirely separate from the other types of backache. Actually,

Pattern Three could just as well be known as Pattern One Plus — that is, a protruding disc plus a pinched nerve. For it is the protruding disc that presses against or "pinches" the nerve. When you know that fact, you won't be surprised to learn that Pattern Three backache exhibits all of the symptoms of Pattern One, along with several of its own. As with Pattern One, Pattern Three comes on over a period of a day or two. The pain builds and stays for weeks. And whenever you bend forward, the pain is worse.

Leg-dominant pain is the hallmark of Pattern Three. Severe pain may radiate to the thigh, calf, or in many cases all the way in to the foot and toes. Typically, a patient with Pattern Three pain will say to me, "My problem is not really my back — it's my leg."

When the diagnosis of a pinched nerve is made, the concern must obviously be whether the pressure is sufficient to damage the nerve's function. In Pattern Three pain, tests of power, reflexes, and sensation are important. Negative results (that is, results indicating that your responses are normal) will support the diagnosis of Pattern One or Pattern Two back pain, or Pattern Three trouble with nerve irritation only. Also, Pattern Four, which we will discuss later in this chapter, seldom produces a continuous loss of nerve function. These four groups make up the great majority of cases, and only rarely will the tests described here show positive findings. If you suspect you have Pattern Three pain, I recommend you try these tests to confirm the nerve's ability to transmit messages. Patients with Pattern One or Pattern Two back pain, or Pattern Four leg pain, may wish to try them as well, since negative results strengthen those diagnoses.

As you set out to take these tests, do your best to adopt an objective attitude about your findings. Try hard not to exaggerate the results in your mind. I know it's impossible to be completely objective and dispassionate about the condition of your own body, but do your best to record your findings as if you were reporting on someone else's condition — some friend whose ailment would cause you to feel concerned but not upset or alarmed.

1. Test your muscle power

This is the most accurate and hence the most significant test you can conduct to determine a loss of nerve function. In Pattern One or Pattern Two back pain, Pattern Four leg pain, or with simple nerve irritation in Pattern Three, you should have normal muscle power. In some circumstances, it may be painful to use that power, but the power should still be there. In other words, don't be misled if your pain inhibits or restricts your movement; that is to be expected. It is quite another thing to find that your muscles will not deliver normal power during these two tests.

A. Can you raise yourself easily to a tiptoe position, that is, up onto the balls of your feet, and back down again? If you're a person of middle age or younger, you will normally be able to raise and lower your heels and arches this way, ten times on both feet at once, and ten times on each foot separately while standing on one leg.

B. Can you walk on your heels? While standing with your feet comfortably apart, raise your toes and arches as high as you can off the floor and see if you can walk that way — that is, with your weight entirely on your heels. It's an awkward gait at the best of times, but, even though it may aggravate your present back pain, you should be able to do this as well as you ever could.

If you can pass both muscular tests, it is unlikely that you have a loss of normal nerve activity.

2. Test the reflexes in your knees and ankles

This is the second most significant of the three groups of tests in this series. The significance of this test depends not on whether your reflexes are strong or weak but rather on whether they have undergone any distinct change, or whether there is a pronounced difference in the reflexes of one leg compared with the other. You may find it much easier to have someone test your reflexes for you.

If you had strong reflexes in the past, before the onset of your back problems, and if you discover now that your reflexes are weak, this could be a significant finding. Or, if you discover that your reflexes are far stronger in one leg than in the other, make a note of this and report it to your doctor when you see him. But, as with the muscular tests, it's the negative results that count most: the normal reactions indicating that you do not have Pattern Three trouble with a loss of nerve function.

A. Test your knee reflexes first — they're easier. Equip yourself with a small, heavy object that will serve as a hammer. A heavy book, say, three-quarters of an inch (2 cm) thick, will do if you use the book's spine as the hammering surface. Sit on a chair of normal height and cross your legs at the knee so that one leg is dangling. Now use your makeshift hammer to strike the soft area of your knee right below the kneecap. It may take two or three tries, but if you do it right, your leg should kick upward in a sudden, involuntary motion. If that well-known knee-jerk reaction occurs, the reflexes in that knee are normal. Now cross your legs in the opposite way and repeat the test on the other knee. Compare this second reaction with the first. If your knee reflexes have been tested this way in the past, consider whether any change has occurred in your reflex ability. If your responses seem about the same for both legs, and if they seem unchanged from your presumably normal past, it is unlikely that you have nerve damage.

B. Test your ankle reflexes in a similar way. In a sitting position, remove your shoes and place the calf of one leg across the other knee, leaving your ankle and foot projecting out to one side, well clear of the opposite thigh. Now perform the same hammering action on the back of your foot, right above the heel — across that cord that most people know as their Achilles' tendon. If you perform this action correctly, your foot should jerk downward. Test both of your ankles this way. If someone is doing this test for you, you should kneel on a chair with your ankles hanging free while the other person taps gently first on one tendon and then on the other. Once you get reactions on both ankles, consider whether they are more or less the same. If they are, again it is unlikely that you have an impaired nerve.

3. Test your legs for sensory ability

This is the least reliable of the three types of tests in this series because feelings are subjective. Whereas muscle and reflex tests produce results that you or your doctor can observe and evaluate, a sensory test relies entirely on your subjective judgment of what you feel.

The idea of this test is to see whether you have experienced any loss of sensation in certain parts of your legs. A loss of sensation is not to be confused with a tingling or "funny feeling" in one or both legs. What we are looking for here is a true inability to feel the split second of pain you normally get from a pinprick in the skin.

To conduct this test, bare your feet and lower legs. Equip yourself with a safety-pin. Seated in any position you find comfortable, reach down and, with a short and rapid jab, prick yourself lightly in the three test areas in succession: first, on the top of the foot in the space between the big and second toe; second, on the top of the foot, just below your little toe; and third, on the calf along the inside of your leg. Repeat this test on the other foot and leg.

If you feel normal pain from each of these locations, it is unlikely that you have a disruption in the nerve's ability to conduct impulses. By deduction, then, your back pain is probably Pattern One, Pattern Two, Pattern Three with only nerve-root irritation, or Pattern Four.

Pattern Four

The leg-dominant pain of Pattern Four is often described as a dull ache. It is not the acute "sciatic" pain so typical of Pattern Three. You might describe your legs as numb, dead, rubbery, or "like blocks of wood." Your symptoms come on with activity — usually just walking for ten or fifteen minutes will do it — and are quickly relieved by rest. But often relief occurs only when you rest in a forward bent position. Slumping in a chair or on a bench may help; standing still and bending forward or squatting down also can reduce your leg symptoms. Many people with Pattern Four leg pain find they can grocery shop for a longer time than they can walk in the mall because in the supermarket they are able to lean forward and support themselves on a shopping cart.

Pattern Four tends to affect older patients. Although each episode comes on rapidly and lasts for only a few minutes, the condition is a chronic one that continues for years and may grow slowly worse.

You may at the same time experience Pattern One or Two back pain, or you may have no backache at all. The nerve's ability to send messages to the legs is normal when you are at rest but can become impaired each time you exercise.

If you have studied the typical stories, conducted the tests carefully, and evaluated the results as objectively as possible, you should now have a good idea whether your back trouble is Pattern One, Two, Three, or Four. Take note that these designations mean what they say: that is, they are *patterns* of back pain, not rankings from "least bad" to "worst."

It may make better cocktail-party conversation to describe yourself as the victim of an acute pinched nerve, the rarest of the four types. But Pattern Three is not necessarily worse than any of the others — it's just different and may require different treatment. While there is no such thing as a "good" kind of backache, each type has its own advantages — if you can call them that — as well as its drawbacks.

Pattern One: Your painful disc may lack the drama of a pinched nerve, but the pain is easier to control. To make things more exciting, you may even indulgently allow friends to refer to your "slipped disc," even though you know by now that discs don't slip. And, incidentally, they don't "disintegrate" either, as you'll see in the next chapter. One drawback to being a Pattern One is the way the pain can linger on as a dull ache. But keep reading. Help is on the way.

Pattern Two: A sore small spinal joint may not gain you much sympathy, even though the pain can be severe at times. At least you have plenty of company in your misery and the chance to swap exotic tales of back pain. And don't underrate the advantage of having a pain that disappears completely between attacks.

Pattern Three: As I pointed out in Chapter One, this is the problem most back sufferers think they have — and most of them, of course, are wrong. You Pattern Threes are an exclusive group. On the other hand, while I would not for a moment make light of your pain, I have to say again that your pinched nerve is not necessarily as painful as it sounds, and it may be less painful than a worn disc or a roughened joint. Just the same, you are more likely to need professional help in bringing your problem under permanent control.

Pattern Four: If you suffer from Pattern Four, probably you are slightly older and able to approach the issue with an air of maturity. At least you are already comfortable at rest, even before you discover the things you can do to improve your exercise tolerance.

Whatever pattern you believe you are, or even if you suspect that you have two, three, or all four patterns at once, take comfort from the fact that positive, gentle stretches and short periods of rest will do wonders for acute back pain and that, thanks to the natural healing process, all bad backs tend to get better with time. Perhaps you will appreciate that last point more fully after you have read the next chapter on the probable causes of common backache.

5   The Causes of Your Back Pain

Now that you have an idea whether you are a Pattern One, Two, Three, or Four pain sufferer, you will want to learn more about the origins of your condition. I've discovered that people who understand the cause of their pain and realize it's not a mystery or beyond comprehension handle the problem more successfully. They are in a position to do something about the pain, to get relief right now.

This chapter is about our current ideas on why backs hurt. But as good as the science may be, these are only theories, our best guess at the source of the pain. What we do know for sure is that backs hurt and that the pain can be classified, as you have already discovered, into four patterns. Except for the few people who require back surgery, our treatment and your control of the problem should be based on those pain patterns, not on the physical abnormality. Where we are sure of the connection, as we must be before an operation, for example, our management can address both areas. If there is any uncertainty about the relationship, we should treat the pattern of pain, not the x-ray, not the test result, not the theory.

Of course, we are all working to improve our knowledge of the causes of your back pain. And we have come a long way. There is strong evidence for the source of each pattern, and that's what we will discuss now.

Let's begin — as your spine itself so often does — with disc trouble. As you recall from Chapter Three, the discs in your spine contain a jelly-like substance that is mostly water. This fluid is being constantly renewed, courtesy of your bloodsteam. Using a chemical reaction, the "jelly" inside the disc absorbs the moisture from small blood vessels nearby. Meanwhile, during the course of a normal day, the weight of your body squeezes some of the moisture out, allowing it to return to the bloodsteam. This cycling process results in the loss of a bit of height while you are up and around. You will regain that height each night as you lie sleeping. If you are young and tall, and if your discs are healthy, you will routinely lose and regain as much as half an inch (1 cm) of height every twenty-four hours. You may have noticed that when you set out to drive home from work in the evening, you have to adjust your rear-view mirror, because you are a little shorter than when you drove to work that morning.

One of the first dramatic demonstrations of this phenomenon took place in 1974, when three U.S. astronauts returned to earth after eighty-four days aboard Skylab, the orbiting space station. To the amazement of their families and the doctors at NASA, the space travelers were each almost 2 inches (5 cm) taller than when they left on the voyage. During those twelve weeks in orbit, their bloodstreams had continued carrying moisture into the discs of their spines; but with no gravity to enforce the other part of the exchange, their discs fattened up with moisture, making their spines longer and the men taller. Once they returned to earth, gravity took over, and within a few hours the astronauts were back to normal size. Since that mission, space suits have been designed to accommodate this stretching of the spine.

Except for those of us who become astronauts, we can all expect to spend our lives, from our teen years onward, permanently losing some of the moisture from our discs. Because of the makeup of the disc's center, the balance gradually fails, and as some people discover, we can lose an inch (2.5 cm) or more in height during our lifetime.

Whenever I describe this process to a group of back patients, somebody always asks why doctors can't do something to replace this lost moisture so as to maintain a person's discs at their original thickness. I point out

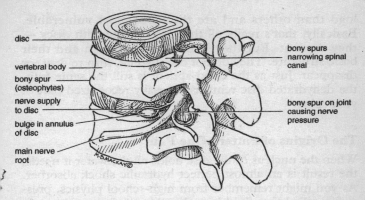

disc

bony spurs
narrowing spinal
canal

vertebral body

bony spur
(osteophytes)

nerve supply
to disc

bony spur on joint
causing nerve
pressure

bulge in annulus
of disc

main nerve
root

M.D.MACKAY©

Fig. 10. A sudden bulge of the disc shell is the probable cause of Pattern 1 pain. Pain is produced by the disc itself and is not the result of pressure on the main nerve.

that this is a natural process we're talking about here — not the onset of a disease. As we will see shortly, the drying-out process within the disc can cause trouble for some people, but in most cases it has the beneficial effect of stabilizing the spine. This is one reason why your back problems are likely to disappear as you grow older.

People also want to know why Nature picks on discs this way, causing them, of all body parts, to lose moisture. The answer to that question is that discs are not exceptional in this respect. Many parts of your body lose moisture as you grow older. Your skin is an obvious example. It's easy to rejuvenate your skin temporarily with a little moisturizer, but we have no way of doing the same thing for your discs. Even a special diet will not alter this natural process.

As the center dries out, the disc flattens like a dehydrated apricot; no longer is it the plumped-up cushion it once was. Some discs in your spine flatten more readily than others, if they are subjected to heavy physical stress. Because of the way your spine is curved, positioned, and structured, a few discs and vertebrae carry more of the load than others and are therefore most vulnerable. Basically, that's really all that goes wrong with discs — they dry out. But they retain their position and their basic structure. They do not disintegrate, turn to dust, or disappear. Just as the dried apricot is still the same fruit, the dehydrated disc remains an easily recognized part of your spine.

The Origins of Pattern One Pain

When the nucleus of the disc holds all the water it needs, the result is an almost perfect hydraulic shock absorber. As you might remember from high-school physics, pressure applied to a fluid in a closed space is spread evenly throughout the container. So pressure on the disc from your body weight or a heavy lift is shared equally around the disc shell, neutralizing the effect. As the disc center begins to dry out, this perfect system starts to fail. The discs begin to narrow — that's the gradual loss of height that comes with aging. The outer shell, called the annulus, bulges out beyond its normal limits. Discs are meant to bulge, its part of the shock-absorber idea, but there is a limit. Finally, the even weight distribution within the disc is destroyed and stress begins to build at a few points under the surface.

The annulus dries out too. Cracks appear, like the cracks in the leather of an old shoe, and the disc wall loses its ability to contain the jelly center. The stage is set for Pattern One backache.

The final event may be dramatic, or the failure may occur with no event at all; in fact, that's usually how it happens. The outer shell gives way; a sudden bulge, then a split or a tear. And the outer portion of the disc feels pain. The same nerve that supplies the back muscles and the small joints and sends messages to the leg provides pain sensation to the annulus. The type of nerve supply the disc receives is the same as the one to the surface of your eye. It can produce a lot of pain.

Sometimes the bulge is gradual and the nerve fibers

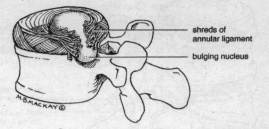

shreds of
annular ligament

bulging nucleus

M.B.MACKAY©

Fig. 11. Protrusion of the disc nucleus usually occurs at the back corner of the disc, a naturally weak area in the outer shell.

have a chance to adjust. The discomfort might be no greater than, say, the gradual bulging of your stomach during a heavy meal. But if the bulge or tear occurs suddenly as the shell gives way, you feel acute pain. As the bulge continues to grow, the pain increases, and this describes the typical onset of Pattern One backache. You have already seen how quickly the pain can spread because of the connections formed by the local spinal nerve: after disc pain comes referred leg pain, then back muscle spasm, then curvature to one side, then additional muscle spasm, and, finally, virtual immobility.

The location of the disc problem accounts for the way Pattern One pain is aggravated when you sit or bend forward. The protruding disc is on the forward side of the pivot point around which you move your spine. It is compressed by any forward motion or by your typical sitting posture. Earlier, I likened the disc to a tap washer being squeezed out of shape under pressure. Bending forward is like tightening down on that tap washer by giving the screw another turn.

The Origins of Pattern Two Pain

The loss of a bit of thickness in a disc — perhaps a quarter-inch (0.5 cm) or less — may not sound like much of a problem. But even that apparently minor loss can mean

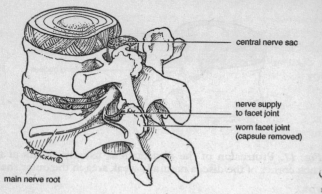

central nerve sac

nerve supply
to facet joint

worn facet joint
(capsule removed)

main nerve root

Fig. 12. Pattern 2 pain appears to result from wear in the small spinal facet joints. The pain signal is trasnmitted to the main nerve root, which is not directly involved.

the difference between comfort and pain. For in addition to its role as a shock absorber, the disc must provide the proper amount of separation between the vertebrae above and below it. Reducing the space between the vertebrae can create wear in the facet joints. If the distance between the bones is decreased, the true alignment of the joints is destroyed. Imagine an electric motor with its central rotor out of alignment. As the motor operates, the misaligned rotor soon begins causing wear among the parts intended to interact with it. Similarly, a facet joint can fall victim to misalignment. As we saw in Chapter Three, the discs of your spine serve as buffers between other parts of your vertebrae but not between the bones of the facet joints. As the disc flattens, the two vertebrae come together and the "unbuffered" bones of the facet joint begin grinding against each other. It's not a pleasant ailment to have, but it's not a disease either — just a local, mechanical problem.

And Pattern Two backache touches off the same ugly sequence of pain radiation that we recited for Pattern One: local pain, leg pain, back muscle spasm.

Meanwhile, at the original trouble spot, the joint becomes inflamed as your body reacts to limit movement and begin repairs. But inflammation produces pain.

At this point, you may become vulnerable to a fearsome little game of Speaking Doctor, because an inflamed joint, as you know now, is called arthritis. For this type of inflammation due to wear, the term is osteoarthritis. It's bad enough to have an inflamed joint, but when it's described as "osteoarthritis of the spine," it sounds like a death sentence. Can't you just visualize your backbone turning to chalk? Yet some doctors, I'm sorry to say, use this term without explaining exactly what it means. If anybody plays this version of Speaking Doctor with you, remind yourself that you do not have a disease. No horrible infection has invaded your spine. When the irritation stops — and it will — the inflammation will clear up and the pain will subside.

Now that you have a clear picture of Pattern Two backache, you can see why the pain is relieved when you bend forward. The forward position removes pressure from those bones at the very back of your spine, and the source of irritation is reduced temporarily. Conversely, any condition that forces you to arch your back — bad posture, pregnancy, a pot belly from being overweight — will increase the pressure and aggravate the pain. Often, these additional conditions are erroneously blamed as the original causes of low back pain. Fat people sometimes slim down in the belief that they can cure their back problems by losing weight. Inevitably they are disappointed, because weight loss, while removing some of the source of aggravation, does nothing to solve the problem of a dry disc or a worn joint.

Posture is very important in both Pattern One and Pattern Two backache. If you are skeptical, try this simple demonstration. In this case, it's your wrist joint we're using as the example. First, make your right hand into a fist and hold it out in front of you with the knuckles facing away. Now, with your left hand, slap hard against the front of that fist. As you'll see, the action causes stress

but no discomfort in your right wrist. Next, open your
fist, straighten out your fingers fully, and arch them back
as far as you can, imitating the way a traffic officer signals
an oncoming car to stop. Now repeat the slapping
motion, forcing the fingers of your right hand back
towards you. Immediately you feel pain in your wrist.
The difference between the two situations illustrates the
difference between force applied to the spine in a balanced posture and force applied when the spine is
already fully loaded. In the first instance, when you
formed a fist, your wrist joint was in "neutral," with
enough "give" to absorb the jolt. In the second instance,
with your fingers bent fully backward, your wrist joint
was held in an extreme position, and the "give" was
gone. The result of the impact was immediate pain. For
the spine with poor posture, the simple act of stepping
boldly off a curb can be enough.

Unfortunately, there is no law to prevent you from
having Pattern One and Pattern Two backache simultaneously or in succession, and if you do, you will display
pain bending both forward and backward, either at the
same time or from one attack to the next, as the case may
be. In fact, I often wonder why that doesn't happen more
often than it does. After all, the same drying action that
allows one side of the disc to bulge leads to a loss of
height and wear in the facet joints. Presto! The One-Two
Combination. Still, for most of us, one pattern clearly
predominates, and that is the pattern that will dictate
treatment.

The Origins of Pattern Three Pain

As if it doesn't cause enough trouble by way of Pattern
One and Pattern Two, the worn disc is also the culprit in
Pattern Three pain — the pinched nerve. Once the center of the disc has lost moisture and allowed the bones to
settle, the outer shell of the disc begins pushing outward.
In this way, it can become directly or indirectly responsible for creating pressure on a nerve.

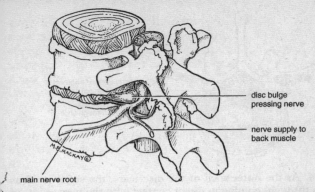

disc bulge
pressing nerve

nerve supply to
back muscle

M.B. MACKAY©

main nerve root

Fig. 13. A bulge at the back corner of the disc that pinches the main nerve root is the likely cause of Pattern 3 pain. Because the root is involved directly, pain is more severe in the leg than in the back.

Before I explain how that happens, I want to interject a word about terminology, in case somebody baffles you by Speaking Doctor about a disc. Throughout this book, I use the expressions "bulging disc" and "protruding disc" as interchangeable terms. I have chosen them because they are readily understood; they do not need to be defined because they are more or less self-explanatory. You may find, however, that your doctor uses some other term to describe the same condition. He may say a disc is herniated, ruptured, prolapsed, cracked, fractured, or distended. They all mean the same thing. Or you may be told that a disc is sequestrated, which means that the bulging has developed to a point where a portion of the disc has torn loose. It's just a further stage of the same process.

As we saw in Chapter Three, one side of each disc is situated very close to the place where a main nerve branch leaves the spinal canal. Once that side of a disc has protruded even slightly, it can easily come into contact with the nerve. And only a slight degree of contact, in the form of touching, rubbing, or squeezing, can be enough to produce pain. That's the direct way in which a

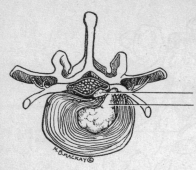

sequestrated fragment
loose in spinal canal

bulging nucleus
tearing through shell

Fig. 14. As the outer shell of the disc tears, the softer nucleus
bulges through, coming in direct contact with the nerve root. In
rare instances, a fragment of the nucleus may break loose and
lie free in the spinal canal.

disc may place pressure on a nerve root. (The disc's indi-
rect involvement in pressure on a nerve is Pattern Four
pain, discussed in the next section.)

When a nerve is pinched by the disc, the problem has
two components. In addition to the unwanted pressure,
the nerve is subjected to a chemical irritation from contact with the disc nucleus. The center of the disc contains a substance that, oddly enough, the body fails to
recognize and therefore tries to eliminate. This attempt
produces a great deal of inflammation and a great deal of
pain. Because the nerve, not the disc or joint, is the principal site of irritation, and because the symptoms follow
the course of the nerve, the leg, not the back, is the principal site of pain.

The sequestrated disc, mentioned a few paragraphs
ago, is fairly rare among people with pinched nerves —
who, in turn, are only a small minority among people
with common backache. Even so, I have seen many cases
of sequestrated discs, and they can be tricky to diagnose.
Once that little piece of disc has torn loose and become
lodged in a nerve canal, a doctor can be confused by the
findings. The disc, having been relieved of the pressure
that caused it to bulge, now emits very little pain. The

severed fragment of disc, having no nerve connections with the body, has no feelings whatever. And the nerve being irritated by the loose piece can exhibit a confusing pattern of symptoms. If the disc is lodged in a nerve tunnel beneath a joint, for instance, the pain will be aggravated when the person arches his back — a symptom of Pattern Two — and yet there will be evidence as well of nerve irritation and leg-dominant pain typical of Pattern Three. When it comes to diagnosis, sequestrated discs are a challenge. They also belong to a small minority of back cases that may require surgery; the quickest way to stop that little piece of wandering disc from making trouble can be to remove it by surgical methods.

Although I have emphasized that the pinched nerve is not necessarily more painful than Pattern One or Pattern Two backache, Pattern Three can certainly cause a lot of leg pain. I have especially vivid recollections of one unfortunate man, a clerical worker in his mid-forties, who swore that the only way he could be comfortable was on his hands and knees.

This man was already in hospital when I first saw him. He insisted on remaining on his hands and knees almost constantly. He stayed in bed on his hands and knees. He took his meals on his hands and knees. He moved to and from the bathroom on his hands and knees. All the staff on the ward regarded him as an eccentric. But, strange as it appeared, examination revealed findings that couldn't be ignored — signs that the man couldn't fake if he tried. Only one conclusion made sense: like many people with Pattern Three leg pain, this man had found he could relieve his pain by arching his back. And because the leg pain was extremely intense, he remained on his hands and knees during every possible moment, allowing gravity to keep his back arched for him. In fact, we found that the man had a protruding disc with nerve pressure — a condition that could be remedied by surgery. We operated, and he was relieved of his Pattern Three pain.

When there is irritation to a nerve, the pain flashes along the length of the nerve branch and all its tributaries. This gives the impression that some of the pain is originating in other parts of the body served by that nerve branch, such as the thighs or lower legs. All four patterns of common back pain can produce leg symptoms, but only Pattern Three, with its mix of acute inflammation and pressure directly on the nerve root, can produce such severe sudden leg pain. This is the only condition that can truly be described as "sciatica." The tests for direct nerve irritation set out in Chapter Four (pages 53-66) are designed to determine whether this is happening.

The Origins of Pattern Four Pain

The fourth pattern of common backache and leg pain is another result of disc narrowing occurring as the disc dries out with age, time, and the effects of everyday living. As the disc flattens and bulges, the adjacent vertebrae come very close together. As we saw earlier, nerve roots leave the spinal canal between every pair of vertebrae. Their points of exit are not holes in the bones but spaces between the bones. When those spaces are reduced, the exiting nerve branch will be pinched. It is the bones, of course, that do the actual pinching, but the disc is the original culprit, for failing to hold the bones apart properly. This narrowing of the spinal canal is often called spinal stenosis, another one of those Doctor words that sounds serious but isn't. "Stenosis" just means narrow, and being told that you have a narrow spinal canal should be about as frightening as being told you have thin hair. And besides, it's not the tight canal itself that is the problem, it's what the lack of space may do to the nerves.

The nerves, just like the other parts of our body, need a normal blood supply. As the vertebrae settle, bony changes occur that begin to interfere with normal blood flow. Bone spurs, called osteophytes, grow along the back edge of the drum-shaped bodies and protrude into the spinal canal. Other bone spurs develop along the sides of the worn facet joints and fill the small exit holes. The nerves are slowly strangled. Usually enough circula-

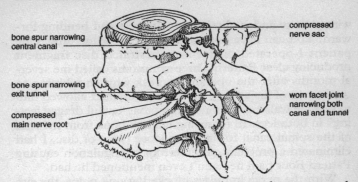

bone spur narrowing
central canal

compressed
nerve sac

bone spur narrowing
exit tunnel

compressed
main nerve root

worn facet joint
narrowing both
canal and tunnel

Fig. 15. Pressure from osteophytes on the central nerve sac and exiting nerve root causes Pattern 4 pain. Leg pain is associated with activity because the pressure prevents adequate blood supply to the nerves.

tion remains to feed the nerves while they are at rest. But the moment the nerves become active, sending messages to your legs as you walk, for example, they need more nourishment and they can't get it.

That's when the leg pain begins. The sensation, an ache or rubbery feeling, is similar to that you might feel if the leg muscles themselves lacked adequate blood supply. It is often relieved when you bend forward because that position opens the exit holes and increases the space within the canal, giving the nerves a chance to recover.

How can you tell whether your pinched nerve (assuming you have one) is the result of direct contact between a disc or a nerve or the result of having a nerve pinched between adjacent vertebrae? The answer is that you may not be able to with certainty. One useful clue is your age. If you are under sixty and have a pinched nerve, chances are the nerve is in direct contact with a disc. If you are older than sixty, it becomes increasingly likely that the nerve is being squeezed between two vertebrae; older people are not usually troubled by newly protruding discs. And the patterns of pain are different. Pattern Three is sudden, severe sciatica made worse with flexion. Pattern Four is a "dead" feeling in the legs that comes on with activity and is eliminated with rest and bending forward. You can have both patterns at the same time. One patient I operated on for a sequestrated disc fragment producing clear Pattern Three symptoms called me several months after the operation to ask why, in addition to getting rid of his acute pain, the surgery had allowed him to resume walking without feeling that "awful draggy feeling" in both legs. In removing enough bone from the roof of the spinal canal to find that loose piece of disc, I had eliminated a problem of nerve-root strangulation causing Pattern Four pain he hadn't even mentioned he had.

With the nerve impulses blocked at one point, the signals are scrambled all along the nerve. The orderly functions of the nerve are disrupted, and the effects are felt right to the boundaries of the system. You lose control of the muscles out there, the responses we call reflexes are blocked off, and you can no longer receive sensory reports from down the line. That is why we were able to say in the previous chapter that you probably don't have Pattern Three pain with an impulse conduction loss if you can pass the muscular test (standing on tiptoe and walking on your heels), the reflex test (knees and ankles), and the sensory test (pricking your calves and both sides of your feet).

Before you drop this book in fright, convinced that you have Pattern Three back trouble about to shut down your entire nervous system, I must make several important points. Not only is Pattern Three — direct pressure on a nerve from a bulging disc — uncommon, but even when it does occur, the pressure is usually so slight that it causes pain from direct nerve irritation without any loss of function. In other words, there is no loss of muscle power, reflexes, or sensation. Finally, in the occasional instance where nerve pressure is long enough and strong enough to disrupt the signals, loss of function happens in only one nerve, supplying, at most, a few muscles or a small area of sensation. The result is serious and may have a profound effect on one movement in the leg or foot, but it can never cause widespread paralysis.

Now, if you have been reading this explanation with a skeptical attitude, you may be saying to yourself, "Well, he makes that sound all very neat and tidy, but how can he assume that the pinched nerve will affect my lower legs and feet? Don't I have other nerve branches running to other parts of my legs and the rest of my body? Couldn't my pinched nerve — assuming I have one — happen to be a nerve that affects, say, my knee or my hip or even my belly button?"

The answer is, yes, it is possible — but unlikely. Again I'm working on the principle that common things happen most commonly.

First of all, as I implied at the beginning of this chapter, as your spine begins to feel the effects of constant use and gradual aging, the spots under heavy stress become particularly vulnerable to trouble. All discs will lose moisture and become flatter, but the real trouble-makers will be the discs that are under heavy mechanical stress.

Back specialists know from experience that, because of the load factor, three discs in your spine are far more likely to cause trouble than all the others combined. One of these is a disc in your neck — the C_{5-6}. It causes problems similar to those that develop in the low back, but only about half as often. Statistically, the great preponderance of trouble comes from two discs in your low back — the L_{4-5} and the L_5-S_1. These are the discs that affect the nerves running into your lower legs and feet — which explains the rationale for the nerve tests in Chapter Four. Those two levels alone account for more than eighty percent of all nerve-root involvement associated with low back pain. And if you include the disc directly above, namely the L_{3-4} (which affects the nerve supplying the knee reflex and the ability to feel on the inside of your calves), we're talking about the sources of more than ninety percent of problems with lumbar discs pressing on nerve roots. In other words, if you have disc problems in your low back affecting your nervous system, there is better than a ninety percent chance that the symptoms will show up in your lower legs and feet.

Now that you know how each of the four patterns of common backache probably develops, see what you can make of this unusual case, which I once had to diagnose and treat.

Scene I: A new patient, a woman I'll call Frances, comes to see me with a familiar story. She has a lingering ache in her low back. The pain is not as acute as it once was, but it has persisted for several weeks. She feels pain as well in her right buttock and down the back of her thigh. By questioning and examining her, I learn that her leg and foot muscles are normal, and so are her knee and ankle reflexes and her ability to sense pain from pinpricks in her calves and feet. When she bends forward, her backache is worse.

What's wrong with Frances? If you remember the descriptions in Chapter Four, you'll have no trouble in identifying her problem as Pattern One backache, the protruding disc.

At the time, I make the diagnosis and prescribe appropriate treatment, and Frances's back pain subsides.

Scene II: Six months later. Frances returns to my office with a new attack of backache. She tells me the old pain reappeared but then disappeared suddenly as a new pain developed in her right calf. In some respects, it sounds like the same old problem, but I soon find significant differences from the last attack. She now has pain the full length of her right leg and into her toes. Her right ankle reflex is gone, and she has lost the ability to feel pinpricks on the outer edge of her foot.

What's going on here? This is a patient who had Pattern One backache, which has disappeared. Everything now points to Pattern Three. Additional testing tends to confirm my suspicions: her Pattern One problem must have ended abruptly because the protruding portion of the disc tore loose, releasing pressure on the disc, just the way a weak spot on a tire will bulge out and then pop. That would account for the sudden cessation of pain. But how do we account for the Pattern Three pain that immediately followed? That fragment of disc that broke free lodged against a nerve and produced Pattern Three symptoms and findings.

The solution? Because Frances doesn't respond to good back care and because her problem keeps getting worse, she enters that small group of back patients who require surgery. In the operating room, I extract that wayward bit of disc from Frances's back. Her problem is solved, and she recovers quickly.

Scene III: Another eighteen months have elapsed. Guess who is in my office again, complaining of terrible back pain. Is it another protruding disc? Another wandering fragment? Neither. Frances presents me with a whole new set of symptoms and findings. By now I know her well enough to believe she is not exaggerating or faking. And so I'm fascinated to check out her condition. Her low back pain is radiating into her buttocks and upper legs. No signs of Pattern Three nerve problems. I rule out the recurrence of Pattern One as well, because bending forward is not especially painful for her. In fact, it seems to relieve the pain. And that's the tipoff: repeatedly arching her back is what hurts most. Frances, having rid herself of Pattern One and Pattern Three backache in that order, has come down with an unmistakable case of Pattern Two!

Now that hardly seems fair, does it? And yet it's easy to understand, once you know the mechanics of common backache. The very same disc that had caused Pattern One pain during its protruding period and Pattern Three during its "wandering fragment" period is now indirectly to blame for the Pattern Two pain. In flattening out, the disc has permitted the adjacent bones of the facet joints to come together and begin grinding painfully against each other.

Fortunately, by the time of this visit, Frances has acquired enough understanding of spinal anatomy to accept my explanation and follow my prescription of proper stretching, strengthening exercises, and improved postural habits. Frances improved rapidly, and as far as I know she is still living normally, free of serious back problems, old or new. If she wasn't I expect I'd be the first to hear about it.

Scene IV: It hasn't happened yet but let's pretend we can see into the future. Twenty years from now, Frances returns with a strange story. Her back is fine aside from the usual aches and pains, but her legs are giving her trouble. When she walks for more than fifteen minutes, they feel full of pins and needles. The problem gets so bad she must stop walking and find a place to sit down. If she slumps forward, a position that makes her feel self-conscious, her leg symptoms disappear within a few minutes. She is ready to start walking and repeat the process all over again.

A new problem? Hardly. It's a typical account of Pattern Four pain, the result of the canal and exit-hole narrowing that followed the flattening of that same old disc. The series of events that caused Frances's Pattern Two backache plus the growth of a few bone spurs over the years have led to constant bony pressure on the nerve roots and a loss of normal circulation.

Her solution may be as simple as a new set of exercises or as dramatic as more surgery, but the problem can be identified and an answer can be found.

As tricky as cases like Frances's can be, they do not support the idea of the back as a medical mystery. I am convinced that any back problem, however complex and puzzling, can be correctly diagnosed and treated. Any back specialist can do it, given the experience, the necessary determination, and full cooperation from the patient.

Mind you, I'm not suggesting that the medical world knows everything there is to know about the human back and what ails it. Certainly there are important facts yet to be determined and questions still to be answered. For instance, what is it about discs that causes them to lose moisture? That is something no one can fully explain. Why do worn joints hurt? Nobody knows. What mechanism of pain operates when a disc touches a nerve? Experiments have proved that pressure alone is not the answer, and we still don't understand all of the chemistry; the full explanation remains to be found. And what about the relationship between wear and mechanical load? Is wear the result of increased activity, or does it just become more significant in active situations? Do the benefits of movement outweigh the damage of constant use? We think so, but again, nobody has all the answers.

My belief is that, as discussed earlier, signs of wear within the spine are a normal development through late middle age. Some years ago, much was made of the fact that soon after farm tractors came equipped with headlights, numerous farmers began suffering from a "new" ailment dubbed "tractor back." Actually, it was just good old common backache created in new circumstances. Headlights had made it possible to plow day and night — twice as long as before. But, in my view, the mere act of sitting on a tractor seat never gave anybody serious back trouble, any more than you could say that the headlights themselves had caused all that back pain. The longer work day simply created unusually prolonged stress, which made normal wear painfully evident.

There is no doubt that certain occupations suffer a higher incidence of back problems. Scientific studies have found a greater than average occurrence of back pain in miners, foundry workers, nurses, stevedores, and heavy equipment operators. The latter group has been studied intensively. There does appear to be a direct relationship between exposure to vibration and the rate a disc ages. The problem lies in trying to place the cart and the horse: what is the cause and what is the effect? Does the increased amount of back pain reflect a real acceleration of the natural aging process from very heavy work, or does work requiring heavy lifting in awkward positions just accentuate normal backache?

One patient I examined who could lay claim to wearing out his back simply through hard work was a blacksmith. Yes, there are still a few blacksmiths around. This

blacksmith was thirty-two years old when I saw him, and
he had been shoeing horses since he was ten. In his adult
years he worked twelve hours a day at his heavy tasks.
Each time he fitted a shoe, he had to bend over at the
waist, hold the weight of the horse's hoof and leg in a
steady position, and swing a heavy hammer. No wonder
his back was sore. He could truthfully say he had worn it
out through hard work. Few of us can make that claim,
no matter what we do for a living or how hard we work.

The encouraging aspect of the story is that even
though he had literally worn out his back, that blacksmith is not prevented from doing anything he wants to
do. Not even his job. Wear in his discs and joints has not
made his work impossible — just more difficult. Like
everyone else with common backache, he can look forward to having his condition improve with age.
Meanwhile, he has cut his work day in half. I put him on
a program of pain control exercise and helped him find
ways of modifying his non-working activities, to give his
back plenty of rest between work sessions.

The real-life case of the blacksmith's backache brings
up two fundamental points — points on which this book
is based. One point is that bad backs tend to repair themselves. As I said earlier, while no one can predict what
will become of any individual's condition as a result of
aging, statistics show that back pain is most common in
the middle years. Backs improve by regaining stability. A
disc will shrink only so far, and then it will become stable
in the new position. Your spine will become shorter;
hence the loss of height as you grow old. Meanwhile,
your spine will grow projections — the bone spurs, or
osteophytes — around a disc, to help stabilize it. In other
words, contrary to popular notion, bone spurs are not
always a source of trouble; rather, they are part of the
solution. It is only in Pattern Four pain where the bone
growths cause a problem. It's almost as if you get too
much of a good thing. Another aspect of the same repair
process is that your facet joints will reshape themselves to
accommodate their new position, eliminating the

increased pressure and allowing room for the nerves to pass by.

The other point is that nearly all the things that need to be done to control your back in the meantime are things you can do for yourself.

Many of my patients are skeptical the first time they are told these facts. They have always assumed that once anybody has a bad back, it will become progressively worse right into old age. Yet, as we all know, as you move into those so-called senior years — from, say, age sixty-five onward — your back stiffens up; everybody's does, whether there has been pain or not. And once your back is less mobile, doing less twisting and bending, its sore spots and weaknesses become less subject to strain. New mechanical back trouble is uncommon after sixty-five. (The elderly are susceptible to backache from some of the causes described in the next sections of this chapter, but these are not mechanical conditions, and they are quite rare.)

My patients have to be convinced as well that the body's marvelous self-repairing process will go to work immediately on any back that is given proper rest. That's hard advice to take, I know, especially when the pain is at its peak; people want something dramatic done for them. But the answer is far less spectacular. It comes in small steps, simple changes in posture that rest the affected area, stretching exercises that reduce the pain, positive adjustments in the daily routine that reduce unnecessary discomfort. It's not magic, but it works, and knowing that can be a great comfort — and a great aid to healing.

The Rarer Causes of Back Pain

Now that I have concentrated so long on the sources, symptoms, and causes of common backache, you may be wondering if I ever concern myself with any other kinds of back pain. The answer is that in my professional work I am concerned with the whole range of back problems.

To cover them all in detail, however, would require a book many times the size of this one, and few readers would find the additional information useful. Such a book would include ailments so rare that not one person in a thousand ever encounters them. Collectively, these diseases account for less than five percent of all back complaints. And even the victims of these rare ailments would gain little from reading about them, for they are generally beyond the realm of self-help. Surprisingly, however, some of the pain associated with these conditions falls into recognizable mechanical patterns and can be dealt with in the same way as the four patterns of common backache we are considering.

If you have symptoms that do not correspond with any that I have described, I suggest that you ask your doctor for a thorough examination. Even if you feel sure that your back trouble is one of the four patterns, you may find it useful to learn a little more about the rarer causes, since you may need to distinguish these from certain conditions of common backache that masquerade under impressive-sounding names such as osteoarthritis of the spine, which, as we saw earlier, is nothing more than an inflamed facet joint.

Here, then, are brief descriptions of some less common forms of backache you may hear about.

Ankylosing Spondylitis

Primarily a young man's disease, ankylosing spondylitis causes widespread acute inflammation of the spinal joints and can also affect the hips, knees, and sacroiliac joints. It is characterized by a visible flattening of the surface of the low back, a loss of chest movement, and marked stiffness of the spine, particularly first thing in the morning. For some reason, ankylosing spondylitis occurs slightly more often in Britain than in North America. As it progresses, the disease stiffens the back by fusing all the vertebrae together. The disease may arrest itself spontaneously at any time.

The pain of the acute inflammation can be relieved by anti-inflammatory drugs. Proper treatment must include instruction in appropriate postural habits, such as sleeping without a pillow so that if the spine becomes fused, it will be fused in its optimum position. Established deformities may require major spinal surgery.

Cancers of the Spine — Primary

These extremely rare diseases may result from cancerous growths in the vertebrae, the bone marrow, the nerves, the muscles, or the fibrous tissues of the spine. Characterized by local tenderness and local pain unaffected by rest or exercise, primary cancer of the spine can usually be detected by blood tests, bone scans, CT, or magnetic resonance imaging.

Any or all of three forms of treatment may be used: drug therapy, radiotherapy (x-ray), and surgery.

Cancers of the Spine — Secondary

Though more common than primary cancers of the spine, these conditions are still relatively rare. The term "secondary" means that the cancer has originated elsewhere in the body, often in the lungs, the breast, or the prostate gland, and then spread to the spine. A person who has back pain as well as cancer in some other part of the body need not assume, however, that the back pain is a symptom of secondary spinal cancer. It is quite possible that ordinary wear, unrelated to the cancer, is causing common backache.

Treatment of secondary cancer of the spine is the same as for primary cancer and can be carried out simultaneously with treatment at the primary site of the disease. Since cancers of the breast and the prostate gland react to hormones, treatment in such cases is likely to involve hormonal therapy.

Osteoporosis

In this condition, which typically occurs in later years, the bones in the back — and the rest of the body, for that matter — become thin. Although the outer diameter and shape of the bones remain the same, the bone mass inside gradually disappears. It is a painless condition that can be considered part of normal aging.

Sometimes, particularly in women after menopause, this loss of normal bone stock becomes extreme and can lead to trouble. Osteoporosis itself does not hurt, but when an abnormally thin bone breaks, it hurts just as much as any other fracture. In the spine, a drum-shaped vertebral body may suddenly give way, often after something as apparently harmless as a cough or sneeze or just missing a step. The fracture will heal and the pain will stop, but multiple fractures can lead to a change in the alignment of the spine with the appearance of the round-shouldered posture stereotypically associated with elderly women.

The resulting mechanical problems are treated like common backache. The best treatment for the osteoporosis is prevention through the formation of strong bones in early life. Once established, osteoporosis is difficult to treat and may be impossible to reverse. Therapies include hormone replacement; specific medications such as fluoride, calcitonin, and parathormone; vitamin D and large-dose calcium treatment, and adopting a lifestyle that excludes smoking and alcohol and includes exercise and a balanced diet.

Paget's Disease

With this affliction, repeated episodes of bone destruction alternate with attempts at normal bone repair. This abnormality can take place anywhere throughout the skeleton, including the back. The effect on the spine may be altered bone growth producing a typical short stature and deformity. Bone may grow into the spinal canal, causing spinal stenosis and pain from chronic nerve compression. The disease is rarely seen before the age of forty.

Rheumatoid Disease

Of all the musculoskeletal diseases affecting people in North America, this is the largest crippler. Definite rheumatoid disease affects one percent of the population, while some features of the disease affect another two percent.

Not everyone with rheumatoid disease has rheumatoid arthritis. The disease has several forms and affects many parts of the body, from the kidneys to the nervous system. We have already learned that "arthritis" means an inflamed joint from any cause, so it is only when rheumatoid disease produces joint inflammation that the condition can accurately be called rheumatoid arthritis.

A person with rheumatoid arthritis will typically suffer inflammation of many joints of the body, including those of the spine. Diagnosis will be confirmed by blood tests and x-rays showing a typical pattern of joint destruction. When the spine is affected, the problem is usually centered in the neck rather than in the low back.

Treatment includes medication ranging from aspirin to gold injections to steroids. General management ranges from instruction in proper rest, exercise, and daily activities to splints and assistive devices. Surgery may be required to repair or replace damaged joints.

According to the American Rheumatism Association, out of every twenty patients with rheumatoid arthritis, five recover completely and five others experience complete healing with residual (but minor) deformities. Only ten percent of patients will have severe joint problems.

Scheuermann's Disease

Some people know this affliction as Juvenile Roundback, so called because its patients, typically between eleven and fourteen years of age, have backs with a pronounced forward curve. This condition results from a defect in the normal growth of the vertebrae, which become wedge-shaped instead of drum-like.

Minor cases can be treated by physiotherapy to improve posture, and, during the growing years, by the application of a brace. Severe cases in adults may rarely require surgery to straighten the spine.

Scoliosis

The most notorious victim of scoliosis, at least in fiction, was Victor Hugo's Hunchback of Notre Dame. Fortunately, few cases of scoliosis are that extreme. A typical case is characterized by an abnormal curve in the spine, a slight hump, and a less obvious protrusion of one side of the chest. The condition, which affects girls more often than boys, begins during adolescence, with the spine twisting and curving to one side. Most scoliosis occurs in the upper back, and although the cause is unknown, we suspect genetic factors play a part. Scoliosis may also result from congenital deformities, accidents, chest surgery, or muscular imbalance caused by paralytic disease.

During growth, a patient can be treated with exercise and bracing. In an adult, severe curves can be corrected only by surgery. Scoliosis affecting the low back may be associated with common backache. The more typical upper back curve is usually pain-free.

About fifteen percent of the population has scoliosis, but most cases are so slight that people are unaware of their condition and no treatment is required.

A different and unrelated form of scoliosis (the term scoliosis applies to any abnormal side-to-side curvature of the spine) occurs in the elderly. In a few people, the natural process of wear is so severe that the back begins to buckle. The process is called degenerative collapsing scoliosis. Rather than the usual symmetrical wear along the spine, the discs and joints become unstable and the lower spine twists into a painful curve. Exercise and posture training can help, but pain control in extreme cases may require surgery.

Spina Bifida

I include spina bifida in this list only because so many people believe it is a cause of back pain. This belief is based on a common misuse of the term, since spina bifida is neither painful nor serious. There is a more extreme form of the same condition, but it is very rare and is known by another name. Early in our embryo stage, the spine and the nervous system are in the form of two flat layers covering the back. As the embryo grows, the layers curve into two tubes, one inside the other. Sometimes the outer tube, which will form the bone, fails to close, leaving a gap through which the inner tube, now the nervous system, is exposed. Extreme cases are obvious at birth because the defect allows the infant's spinal cord and nerves to protrude under the skin. This condition is called meningomyelocoele. The harmless minor form of this problem, termed spina bifida, typically involves only one vertebra, with a gap in its posterior elements so narrow — 1 or 2 mm — that its existence is discovered by chance, years later, when the spine is x-rayed for some other reason. The gap is full of thick, fibrous tissue, and the spine is functionally normal. This minor x-ray defect is not a cause of back pain.

Spondylitis

Spondylitis is an inflammatory condition of the spine, which may arise from an infection or chemical reaction. If it is produced by a bacterial infection, it is sometimes called osteomyelitis of the spine. Chemical irritation may occur as a result of tests, such as discography, conducted to diagnose back pain. Infection may result from surgery, open back injury, or an infection that spreads to the spine from elsewhere in the body.

Whatever the source of trouble, the inflammation/infection is usually treated with antibiotics, rest, and sometimes a brace or cast to immobilize the spine. Rarely, surgery will be undertaken to drain the infection or decompress or fuse the affected segment.

Spondylolisthesis

This is not a disease but a mechanical condition in which one vertebra slips over another. Discs never slip, but oddly enough the bones sometimes do. This may happen for any of five reasons: a defect within the interlocking joint system at the back of the spine (a condition called spondylolysis, which is described next); a congenital abnormality in the design of a facet joint; an advanced case of wear in a set of facet joints; a major trauma; or a bone ailment, such as Paget's disease, which changes the shape of the bone.

In adolescents, surgery may be required to restore the vertebra to its proper position. In adults, minor cases of spondylolisthesis are treated like common backache. Severe slips may require surgery to control the associated patterns of pain.

Degenerative spondylolisthesis caused by severe wear in a pair of facet joints is a local version of the degenerative collapsing scoliosis I have already described. For unexplained reasons, the degenerative slip occurs most often in women over the age of forty-five at the L_{4-5} level. The pain is a combination of Patterns One, Two, and Four. And as with the collapsing scoliosis, surgery may be required to eliminate the pressure on the nerves and control the back pain.

Spondylolysis

Not to be confused with spondylolisthesis — though it often is, even by doctors — spondylolysis is a defect in the posterior portion of a vertebra, usually one in the low back. Although its cause is not certain, it is thought to result from a fracture in early childhood (before age five), that fails to heal. The result is an abnormal separation between the upper and lower sets of vertebral joints. Intermittent back pain is the typical symptom. Although spondylolysis may cause slippage of the affected vertebra (spondylolisthesis), this complication is by no means inevitable. Nor does the unmended break necessarily

cause common backache. The incidence of spondylolysis
in the population at large is about ten percent. Among
the Inuit of Baffin Island, in the Canadian Arctic, the
incidence is fifty percent, perhaps because youngsters
there are habitually falling on the ice.

Throughout this book I am assuming that you, the reader, have none of the rare afflictions listed here but are
suffering instead from common backache. It's a reasonably safe assumption, and if it's correct, I can assure you
that not only have you a lot of company but also you are
one of the lucky ones — if anyone with back pain can be
called lucky. For while it is not my intention to dissuade
anyone from seeing a doctor, I want to make it clear to
you that the self-help procedures set out in this book may
be all the treatment and therapy you will need to bring
your back trouble under control for the rest of your life.

6 *Is It All in Your Head?*

I have seen unusual back patients in my day but none more bizarre than a man I'll call Ralph.

In his late thirties, Ralph suffered from common backache, which he relieved by lying in bed day after day. Nothing bizarre about that. But Ralph, you see, was a professional writer, and by the time I saw him he had become obsessed with his problem and with the need to go right on working in bed — word processor and all. He had designed and built an elaborate frame on which he suspended his word processor over his bed so that he could somehow manage to write while flat on his back.

Although I never saw his contraption, I could tell by the way he described it that he had put a great deal of thought and effort into its design and construction. If he had devoted even half as much time and energy to back exercise and care, he could have been leading a normal life by this time, with little or no pain.

Obviously, that was not what he wanted. He was inordinately proud of his invention and content with his self-appointed role as a bedridden martyr with an incurable illness.

I don't know why Ralph came to see me, unless it was to gain medical approval of his ridiculous "solution" to a routine problem. In any case, the moment I suggested a more rational approach, I lost him as a patient. I never saw him again, but he has remained in my memory as one extraordinary example of how a person's emotional response to back trouble can shut out any attempt at sensible treatment.

Even among back patients who respond more moderately to pain than Ralph did, there is always an important emotional element that must be considered along with the physical. Previous chapters have offered a thorough grounding in the physical aspects. Now it's time to gain a clear understanding of the role your emotions play in making your back ache.

Most people, I think, recognize that there is a close relationship between mind and body. They know, for instance, that physical illness can readily cause an emotional upset, and that a positive emotional response can play an important role in warding off an illness or bringing about a speedy recovery. But I have found that many people with back problems do not realize, or will not acknowledge, the extent to which their emotions can contribute to their pain.

When you feel a twinge of back pain, your first reaction may be physical, in the form of muscle spasm. Or it may be emotional, in the form of anxiety or fear. The nature of your emotional response depends upon your personality, but regardless of the type of person you are, there is always a response. Chronic back pain is never just a physical problem. Your emotional response, though not necessarily thought out in words, may amount to something as simple and obvious as, "Look out — here comes a new attack of back pain!" That emotion, in turn, will trigger a muscle spasm, which produces pain. The pain triggers more muscle spasms and more anxiety. And so it goes — not around in a circle but in a downward spiral, with the physical and emotional elements becoming more intense at each round.

This pattern is not peculiar to backache, by any means. Worry can aggravate almost any physical illness, and vice versa. Feelings of depression are a common reaction to heart problems, for instance, and they can be so inhibiting to recovery that some heart specialists refuse to risk surgery while a patient's morale is low. I am convinced, however, that the emotional element is even more destructive in back pain than in other illnesses because those myths and misconceptions we discussed in Chapter One generate fears and anxieties far out of proportion to the actual physical problem. Such emotions can become powerful and destructive forces in our lives — if we let them.

Emotion can cause physical illnesses, or emotion can determine our reaction to illness from a different, purely physical source. Witness our bedridden friend with the word processor. Emotion can influence the way we follow a doctor's advice. ("He told me to get up on the second day, but I was afraid of hurting my back again. So I stayed in bed for the rest of the month.") Emotions can prolong our symptoms. I have many patients whose bodies have memorized old pain and continue feeling it long after the original physical condition has ceased to be the cause.

Emotional tension can bring on an attack identical to the original physical episode. I can testify to that phenomenon from personal experience. Several years ago, I was teaching my young daughter how to do somersaults. I discovered it is impossible to describe a somersault to a six-year-old and expect to be understood. I had to perform a demonstration. In the course of doing just two somersaults, I wrenched my neck and developed an acute Pattern Two pain. The pain subsided rapidly, as I expected, and I had forgotten the episode when, three months later, I was performing a very difficult operation. As the tension mounted, the neck pain suddenly reappeared. It was identical to the pain I had suffered while somersaulting. I hadn't reinjured my neck: I was just suffering emotional tension. The moment the operation ended — successfully — my neck pain disappeared. I had experienced a textbook example of memorized pain.

The key to controlling negative emotions is understanding. Without knowing you personally, I could not predict your emotional reactions to backache — or any other illness — because we all respond in our own way. When two people suffer broken legs, one may go into a state of depression and stare at the wall for hours, while

he other uses the enforced spare time to call old friends
or catch up on some reading. There are, however, certain
nteractions of mind and body that are common to us all,
and by understanding them you can begin to explore
your individual emotional responses to backache.

First, let's see how emotional stress can aggravate
physical pain. This can happen in three ways, which I
sum up as "tension," "focus," and "body language."

Tension is a normal condition; your muscles couldn't
function without it. But sometimes it occurs for emotional reasons. If those emotional feelings remain unex-
pressed and unreleased, the tension persists. Prolonged
tension produces pain.

Suppose, for example, that you have an argument with
your spouse at breakfast. You become angry. Your stomach churns. Your jaws clench. The muscles in your neck,
shoulders, and back tighten up. That tension may remain
throughout the day. By late afternoon you may have forgotten all about the argument, but your body hasn't. And
that tension is now producing pain. An early-morning
argument has become literally a pain in the neck and you
don't even realize the connection. If you happen to be
one of the millions of people with mechanical back problems, you have already discovered that poor posture and
specific movements can lead to backache and muscle
spasm. You are about to discover that the reverse is also
true. Your muscular tension can produce pain at the site
of mechanical problems. The cycle runs both ways and
you could be in for a dandy bout of back pain.

Focus is the term many of us use to describe the
process of concentration. Our minds routinely screen out
many impulses that constantly bombard our senses. This
enables us to concentrate on whatever is important to us
at the moment. If you are sitting at a public meeting, listening to a good speaker at the front of the hall, your
mind will focus your attention so that you become obliv-
ious to the hardness of the auditorium chair, the hum-
ming of the ventilation system, the glare of the ceiling
lights, or the whiff of cologne behind you. If the speaker

is very good, your focus may be so strong that almost nothing will disrupt your concentration. That's a useful form of focus.

Sometimes, however, we are inclined to focus our attention on pain. Soon we become conscious of it to the exclusion of everything else. It's like running your tongue over a tooth cavity, even when you know the action will hurt. The more we focus on pain, the more we feel it. And pain is a spell-binding speaker.

You can avoid this hazard by adopting techniques set out in a later chapter of this book — exercises and postural habits that become second nature and pleasant substitutes for the destructive practice of focusing on pain. That's one of the key elements in controlling pain-focused behavior: concentrate on something else. It sounds too simple to be the answer, but it is an essential first step in conquering the problem.

Body language is an unconscious means we all use to express feelings we can't put into words. Watch somebody as she unconsciously nods her head as she listens to a person with whom she agrees. Notice the erect, shoulder-back posture of the man who just got the raise he knew he deserved. Observe the dejected slump of the clerk at his desk who has just been told that after a week's effort the accounts don't balance. These are all instances of body language that everybody can recognize.

A homemaker has a rough day at home with the children. Her husband comes home and sits down to read the paper. She feels a strong need to tell somebody how tired and discouraged she is, but he doesn't seem interested. She decides not to bring up the subject. As she represses her feelings, her body begins expressing them for her. She sticks her chin out in a defiant pose and clenches her fists. She tenses her shoulders as she literally "gets her back up." Although she doesn't realize what's happening, she's finding another way, through her body, of saying, "Hey — I've had a bad day." If, like so many of us, she suffers mechanical neck pain, the muscles in that area will already be accustomed to reacting with spasm, and the reaction to her repressed hostility will produce the same painful response. Here is another important point: the pain from a non-mechanical source is just as painful and just as real as the pain from one of the four patterns of common backache. Had this woman realized how the repression of her feelings would affect her, she would probably have made the effort to express those feelings directly.

Body language can produce pain, usually neck pain, in a different way. Remember our dejected clerk? As he sits at his desk pondering his hours of wasted work, his shoulders slump and his head pushes forward. Suddenly he has neck pain rapidly rising to become a headache. Muscle tension? Suppressed hostility? Depression? It's none of these; it's poor posture. Holding his neck in a forward bent position is a good way, as you now know, to produce Pattern One pain. Of course his emotional state will intensify the pain, but the real source is just mechanical strain.

Physical pain is capable of generating a wide range of emotional responses. An attack of back pain, especially, can generate fear, anxiety, panic, hysteria, despair, depression, frustration, hopelessness, guilt, inadequacy, a sense of failure — or almost any combination of these emotions.

Not long ago I examined a man who had already been referred to physiotherapy by his family doctor. By his manner and the expression on his face I could see that he was frightened out of his wits. When I asked him what was bothering him, he showed me a slip of paper he had in his wallet. It was the requisition his doctor had made out for the physiotherapist. The man had just spent a considerable amount of time listening to his doctor describe what he had found wrong with the man's back. Throughout the explanation, the doctor had emphasized repeatedly that the problem was not serious and was not a disease. But when the patient read the requisition, he found a term that seemed to contradict everything the doctor had said. It read "osteoarthritis." One fearful and misleading phrase from the physician had been enough to touch off an emotional reaction that damaged the patient's morale — and aggravated his back pain.

A more typical story is the woman who arrived at one of the Canadian Back Institute locations in a bad state of fright. Her doctor had told her she had several slipped discs. She believed that any violent movement could cause her spine to collapse into a pile of bones. I'm sure that until she learned the facts about her condition, that poor woman suffered more from fear than from backache.

One emotional response often generates many others. A fearful person may grow panicky and withdraw from all activity: no work, no recreation, no sexual relations. In the extreme, the person may suffer financially and socially, with less income and few associations with friends — conditions that touch off feelings of inadequacy, loneliness, self-doubt, and concern over money. Sexual problems produce feelings of insufficiency on the part of the backache victim, resentment on the part of the partner, and frustration for both.

Severe emotional responses may not be triggered by a single acute attack, but they are almost inevitable with chronic trouble, by which I mean either a persistent backache or a series of repeated attacks with perhaps only short periods of relief between them. Chronic backache is especially conducive to depression because the pain gives you the feeling that your normal life is over and that you will be suffering this way for the rest of your days.

The difference between a manageable attack and an unmanageable chronic condition is like the difference between physical punishment and random torture. A person sentenced to a clearly defined form of corporal punishment can brace himself for it, endure it, and begin to recover. The agony is a thousand times worse for the prisoner who has no idea when the goons will show up at his cell door, how severe the next session will be, or how long it will last. Worst of all, he can't help fearing that his ordeal will go on for the rest of his life. You may identify readily with that second situation if the back-pain goons have been at your door.

There is no need, of course, for you to undergo such psychological torture. You can learn to live with your condition without having to live with the pain or suffer the anticipation of a severe attack. It's within your power to banish virtually all those emotional responses by learning to cope with any attack of pain. Once you get to know your back and understand how resistant it is to real damage, and once you master the techniques of relieving the acute pains that may occur, you are on your way to winning the psychological side of the battle.

Before you enter the fray, it's wise to know your enemy. Begin by separating chronic pain, which is pain of long duration, from chronic-pain behavior, an abnormal lifestyle in which pain becomes the constant center of attention and the basis for all activity. I remember one woman, let's call her Clare, who was totally unaware that pain had taken over her life. She told me proudly that, in spite of her symptoms, she had continued her favorite hobby, gardening. Of course, her pain would allow her to work for only a few minutes at a time but she had solved that problem. None of her flower beds were larger than a couple of feet in diameter. She could tend one, then lie on the ground and rest before crawling to the next. I never got to see Clare's strange garden, but even without that first-hand inspection, it was clear that her pain not only ruled her life, it ruled her landscape.

You might counter, at least she wasn't bedridden. True, but she wasn't at work either, and except for her garden of agony, she had no interests, no hobbies, and no hope for the future. Clare was a prisoner of her pain behavior, and her garden was a proud pain-focused symbol of her plight.

Clare illustrates another point. It is not easy to identify pain behavior, especially in yourself. There are clues, but no single characteristic marks an individual as dominated by pain. Taken together, however, a pattern begins to emerge, a pattern as well-defined as the mechanical pain patterns I have already described. At CBI we have come to call this collection of symptoms Pattern Five.

Pain behavior develops over time; six months is the classic period. Of course, it can begin more quickly. There is usually a diagnosis of "soft tissue injury" or some other vague description reflecting the doctor's inability to find a physical cause for the problem. The physical examination is inconclusive, and a battery of tests and x-rays has failed to identify the source of the pain. Many doctors are consulted and many treatments tried without success.

In almost every case, the pain-focused patient has difficulty sleeping, suffers from an expanding array of unrelated symptoms, endures sexual dysfunction, and clings tenaciously to the belief that an obscure and undiagnosed physical problem is the basis for all the trouble. The total rejection of a behavioral abnormality as a possible source closes the door on the best route to recovery.

Pain-directed behavior is never active behavior, and prolonged inactivity leads to the real physical problems of poor muscle tone, joint stiffness, and loss of fitness. Often, this lifestyle is encouraged accidentally by the way you and your family interact. Your family may do you — and themselves — a disservice by showing either too much concern about your back problems or too little.

Over-concern, ironically, is a big danger for the person who is the ever-reliable "pillar of the family." I sometimes describe it as the Iron Homemaker Syndrome, because it so often affects wives and mothers who have spent years serving their families without letup — never sick, never taking a day off, always on hand to cook the turkey on Thanksgiving, always the one who cleans up the mess afterward.

Homemakers, of course, are not the only ones who find themselves in situations of this kind. This phenomenon affects people of both sexes. I think of it as the Iron Homemaker Syndrome because it is imposed most often upon females who are the "anchors" of their households. Marriage and sex have little to do with it except that they

are part of the circumstances in which a person is expected to behave as though she were indestructible. Cast in
this role, anyone — male or female, married or unmar-
ried — is likely to respond in the same way to a sudden
attack of back pain. The attack may be entirely physical
at the onset, but the Iron Homemaker immediately has a
new need: the need to express her fear of what's wrong.
Yet she has never felt comfortable showing any weakness.
She can't talk about this feeling and she can't dismiss it.
Her solution, to the surprise and alarm of her family, is
to collapse into complete immobility.

The family rallies around her, convinced that whatever
is wrong must be terribly serious because Good Old
Mother would never let a minor back ailment slow her
down. Now Mother is on the spot. Subconsciously she
has to live up to her family's new expectations. The only
way to do that is to suffer intense pain. Can you think of
a more unpleasant way to get that message across?

As a back doctor, I often have great difficulty with this
all-too-common occurrence, because I'm faced with the
task of trying to make Mother and her family understand
the real source of her backache. Certainly her problem is
physical — or at least it was at the beginning. But I have
to convince everyone that the major, lasting disability is
largely emotional.

"Never!" says the family. "Mother has always been the
best worker we know. Magnifying her problem?
Rubbish!"

Usually my comments are interpreted to mean that
Mother is mentally unbalanced and that I am dismissing
her pain as unreal.

Of course the pain is real. No one, least of all someone
who is familiar with back pain, would ever suggest that
the pain isn't real, or that it isn't as intense as Mother
and her family say it is. Mother isn't a liar and she isn't
faking the attacks. But the problem is not in her back as
much as in her body's unexpected and devastating
response to the pain. I always find that a hard message to
get across, especially to a family convinced that either I

don't understand the seriousness of the problem or I have no compassion for the stricken patient.

Ironically, the same emotional response — subconsciously intensified pain — can occur if a family displays too little concern for a backache victim's problems. When back pain strikes, the victim needs attention. If the family seems indifferent, the victim may be too considerate or too proud to demand attention in so many words. And so the body makes the demand instead, by producing a convincing degree of pain. The message is, "See, I really am in agony. Now everyone has to notice me."

Like everyone else, you could be the victim of over-concern or under-concern on the part of the people around you — and not necessarily your family. It could happen to you at work. If you have been playing the role of Reliable Charlie — never late, never off sick, always there when needed — you may have set yourself up as a victim of over-concern on the part of your colleagues. Or, if your role is less conspicuous, you could suffer indifference from the people at work. Either way, your back pain will undergo some unnecessary aggravation.

Both situations can lead to the same reaction. As you subconsciously prolong your pain, your family or colleagues grow suspicious: "Are you sure it isn't all in your head?" By now, there is no way that words can prove what you know is true. The only convincing response must come from your body — in the production of more pain. Your body can't allow you to get well without making you look like a phony.

You have to remember that these reactions take place outside your conscious control. Your mind and your back simply gang up on you to get what they want — more attention, more rest, more help. But you pay the price in continuing back pain.

As you have probably surmised by now, you can avoid the hazards of over-concern and under-concern by understanding these emotional processes in advance. Once you are aware of the problem, you can seek a solution. What are the circumstances that surround and perhaps feed your pain? Is your pain a means to control events that are otherwise unmanageable? Is a need for affection or attention a factor? Is pain your escape from an intolerable situation? Are you financially dependent on your pain? It's difficult to be objective about such personal questions, but without honest answers in the privacy of your own mind, you can't even begin to recover.

What we're talking about here, essentially, is the danger of becoming dependent upon your pain. If you allow this to happen, your pain can become an indispensable part of your life. Dependency on illness, and on pain itself as proof of that illness, figures all too often in the lives of back patients who could otherwise recover swiftly. It happens, often undetected, in private relationships, and it happens more visibly — at least from my vantage point — to people who claim workers' compensation or accident insurance payments, or who enter into litigation over back injuries.

One situation I know involves a patient of mine, a young man who lives with a middle-aged woman. The woman provides him not only with room and board but also with the support and sense of family he was denied as a boy. Why is she so solicitous? The poor young man has a bad back. As long as his back continues to produce pain, he has a meal ticket and the freedom to come and go as he pleases. He is paying a heavy price in pain, but you can imagine how he would resist any effort to make his back feel better.

I have another patient who sees himself as a superjock. He insists he was on his way to becoming a professional hockey star until he developed back trouble. This man truly believes that only because of his back did he fail to achieve a career as a successful athlete. Actually, my patient tried out for the team he wanted to join, couldn't make the grade, and then developed back trouble. Now he's stuck with back pain as his permanent excuse for not being another Wayne Gretzky.

You may think these people are malingering — that is, lying — but I can assure you they are not. I have examined these two young men, and many others like them, and I know their pain is real. It may not arise in their discs or facet joints, but by the time it registers in their consciousness as back pain, it hurts just the same.

The difference between malingering and using real pain in role playing is the difference between telling a lie and living an unhappy truth. I like to illustrate that important difference with the analogy of the flooded basement. Suppose an acquaintance calls up and wants to come over to your house. You don't want him to visit but you are too polite to say so. Instead, you make up an excuse; you tell him you're in a crisis — the basement is flooded. You're lying, but you expect to get away with that story. That's malingering. Now suppose, instead, that you tell the same story and then feel compelled to hurry downstairs and flood your basement, just to make your story true. That, in effect, is what your subconscious does when it uses back pain to enable you to play a role. The big drawback, of course, is that you now have to cope with that basement full of water — or live with that aching back.

Sometimes, especially when money is involved, people in positions of authority may encourage you to maintain your dependence on your pain. If you are involved in litigation over a back injury, this may be done inadvertently, in the normal course of preparing your case. Your lawyer will call you up from time to time and ask, "How's your back?" You may not have thought about your back for weeks, but now he has made you focus on it. Even more insidious is the use of a pain diary. You are asked to keep close track of your pain and write down every episode with exact time and intensity. The idea is to convince the court that you are severely disabled. Of course, the person who becomes really convinced is you. And since you are going to court over it, you are not about to embarrass your lawyer or yourself by getting well too soon. The last thing you are likely to say is, "Drop that case — my back is all better." Yet, medically speaking, that might be the smartest thing you could do.

A lawyer might also encourage you to prolong your pain as a cautionary measure: "We don't want to settle until you're completely well." Now, when was the last time you were ever completely well, with not so much as a twinge of pain or a stiff joint anywhere? Advice like that may be smart law, but it's bad medicine.

Compensation boards and accident insurance schemes can be even more blatant about encouraging you to cultivate your back pain. That's not what they intend to do, but occasionally the system seems to operate that way. Instead of motivating you to recover and return to work, the system rewards you for feeling pain and punishes you for getting well.

If you have ever filed a claim for compensation or accident insurance, you will probably identify readily with the man in this next story, even if your job and personal circumstances are different from his. This man is a poorly educated immigrant who digs ditches for a living. He is hard at work one summer morning when he wrenches his back. Quite properly, he quits working and claims compensation from a government-operated board and accident insurance from a fund supported by his employer.

His sore back keeps him off the job for six months, and the payments he receives make it possible for him to visit his sunny native land. He spends four months there, visiting with old friends and relatives. Shortly before Christmas he returns home feeling much better and decides to go back to work in the new year. On the second day of January he pulls himself out of bed at 6 a.m. and rejoins his work crew. It's still dark outside. The weather is cold and snowy. The ground is frozen. The moment he puts shovel to earth, his back pain hits him again. Maybe you can think of several reasons why he should keep right on working, but at this moment he can't think of any. On the contrary, he can find at least four reasons why he'd be far better off if he went back on the sick list:

1. After four months of vacationing in the sunshine, who needs cold winds, snow, and frozen ground? And

the man is not malingering. He's reacting normally. How great do you feel on the first day after your vacation, when you have to pry yourself out of bed and get back to work? Try getting back into harness after six months of nothing to do.

2. His back is sore again. And no wonder. Six months' idleness has left his physique in bad shape, and yet he feels he must prove he's as good a ditch digger as ever. Nobody has shown him there are ways of digging that will protect his back against unnecessary strain. What's worse, this is the first back pain he's felt in three months.

3. He's convinced that with every bit of pain he feels, he is causing permanent new damage to his back. Nobody has told him what's wrong with his spine. It's only a simple case of Pattern One back pain aggravated by the strain of bending forward and digging, but he doesn't know that hurt is not the same as harm.

4. Financially speaking, he's crazy to be working again when he could be collecting benefits. Since his workers' compensation and his insurance benefits are both tax-free, he was pocketing more money while he was idle than he normally takes home in wages, after taxes, for mucking around in a half-frozen ditch. He has taken a cut in pay to come back to work.

Put yourself in his place. What would you do in those circumstances?

Your answer will depend on what you want out of life. I've thought a lot about that question, and I think that if I felt the way that ditch digger feels — and if I had as many misconceptions as he has about back pain — I'd probably walk right off the job and go back on compensation.

The only trouble with my decision is that I would be stuck with the back pain. If I got better, I'd have to go back to work, and the whole cycle would start over again. But how long could I nurture my back pain? And what would I do when the back pain had become my sole occupation and the compensation benefits had run out? I couldn't afford to be in pain for nothing, but I would be forced to do that — or go back to work.

I can't predict what your decision would be in those circumstances. But one basic purpose of this book is to point out the temptations and pitfalls of becoming a "professional" victim of back pain. No one suffering chronic back pain wants to stay that way. Without exception they tell me, "All I want to do is get better and go back to work." In one sense they do, but only on their own terms after I or some other back specialist have cured their problem and returned them to normal.

The reality is quite different. There is no cure and there is nothing that I or any of my colleagues can do until the patient is willing to take an active role and, more important, take responsibility.

If you are in the grips of pain behavior, getting free can be one of the most difficult things you have ever done. Begin by shifting your focus to something other than pain. You can't just forget it; something must take its place. Imagine a beautiful field of lush grass under a warm summer sky. In the middle of the field is a small hill and on the hill stands a magnificent white horse. Close your eyes and study the picture. Now, do it again, but without the horse. Just the field and the hill, no horse. Don't think about the horse. You see; it can't be done. The more you don't think about the horse, the more majestic he becomes. Consider that the next time someone tells you not to think about your pain.

Now picture the same field and hill with a large gray elephant standing on the knoll. Suddenly that other animal (what was it again?) is gone. You have changed your focus.

Set physical goals that are not related to pain. Focus on how far you can walk, how long you can sit or how much you can lift. Your target must be both measurable and achievable. Start at a level of activity you can tolerate, no matter how little that may be, and gradually increase your function until you reach the chosen goal. Keep a careful record of your progress, a diary of achievement, not of pain.

At the Back Institute we have learned that pain remains or even increases while ability improves. But pain is no longer our focus. We accept the pain as real and inevitable, but our goal is function — and that's what we measure. For the patients who escape chronic pain, the change often comes suddenly. Somehow your body recognizes that your increased level of activity is not compatible with your perceived level of pain, and the pain gives way.

Putting you on that road with the chance of success is the best anyone can do. The rest is up to you.

7 Can a Chiropractor Help?

Sooner or later, many people with low back pain give up on their doctors and turn elsewhere for help.

Typically, they will visit chiropractors or other practitioners whose theories and techniques lie somewhere on the fringe of conventional medicine. Some patients, perhaps those who are well-to-do, but even some who are not, may be inclined to travel to a distant spot on the globe for treatments at expensive clinics or spas. Whatever treatment they choose, a few people come away feeling better than they have in years. But others end up more discouraged than ever, often suffering continuing pain, disappointment, and unnecessary expense.

Anyone who is disenchanted with conventional doctors will have no trouble finding promising alternatives — osteopaths, chiropractors, homeopaths, herbalists, reflexologists, and various others. Osteopaths may resent being included in this group, since they enjoy the status of doctors in several parts of the world, including the United States. Nevertheless, osteopathy does represent an alternative to conventional medicine and, from what I know of their training and work, osteopaths place a greater emphasis on manipulation than the typical medical practitioner. In their scope of practice, however, the osteopath is in most respects similar to the family doctor. With further training, osteopaths can be licensed to perform surgery.

Over the past thirty years, acupuncturists and acupuncture have gained a place in back pain management throughout North America. There is no doubt that acupuncture can be effective in the early management of some acute pain, but its continued use for a chronic back condition is completely unjustified. What's more, this approach to simple drug-free pain control has spawned a host of imitators with even less apparent value. Electric or laser acupuncture and acupressure are unproven treatments that can distract back pain sufferers from remedies that are less dramatic but of greater established value.

As far as some North Americans are concerned, acupuncture was "discovered" in the early 1970s by James Reston of the *New York Times*. On assignment in the Orient, Reston had his appendix removed by Chinese doctors using acupuncture instead of anesthetic. As any reporter would, Reston wrote about the experience in full detail. Almost overnight the ancient art of acupuncture became the latest North American fad. Ironically, with the continued cultural exchange between Far East and West, Chinese doctors have made a similar "discovery" of our methods of modern anesthesia and many have come to regard acupuncture as passé.

My own view of acupuncture is that it represents one way of providing short-term relief from transient, acute pain. This raises an important point that is often misunderstood. Acupuncture is only a method of pain relief. No one who practices acupuncture in an honest and scientific manner will claim that it cures anything, in the sense of solving a structural problem or bringing about a physical improvement.

The needles used in acupuncture apparently trigger the body's production of those hormones called endorphins, which are natural opiates, or pain-killers, comparable to morphine. The existence of endorphins was discovered only in the mid-1970s, and nobody can say at this point where that discovery will eventually lead. What can be said is that no one has yet shown acupuncture to be useful in the long-term treatment of sore backs.

Speaking more generally, I am automatically skeptical of any approach that suggests that common backache can be permanently relieved, let alone cured, by any single form of treatment. It is one thing to say, as I do, that the natural healing of any form of common back trouble will be assisted by the temporary avoidance of painful activities, gentle exercise, and proper postural habits. It is quite another to claim that manipulation or mineral baths or herbs or injections of some kind will restore your spine to health, regardless of whether you have a painful disc, a worn facet joint, or a pinched nerve. There is nothing mysterious about common back pain, but it can be complicated, and its various forms obviously require a variety of treatments.

Apart from their handicap of "tunnel vision" about treatment, practitioners who offer alternatives to conventional medicine often lack many of the skills and most of the resources that a good back doctor uses in his work. Osteopaths in the United States are exceptions in this respect, but chiropractors are not. Unlike members of the established medical community, few chiropractors have access to pathology departments or surgical experience. They are not party to recognized medical research or privy to its results. They're out there somewhere, all alone with their theories, among colleagues who can offer little of the stimulation — call it "cross-pollination" — that occurs when conventional exponents of various specialties consult under one hospital roof.

Chiropractors presume to diagnose spinal problems as well as treat them, and yet in many cases their use of x-rays is misleading and their concept of spinal anatomy is remarkably unscientific. I know of one chiropractor who has been using manipulation of a patient's neck in an attempt to straighten her crossed eyes. Yet there is no connection between the movement of the eyes and the nerves or muscles of the neck.

Some chiropractors also treat children suffering middle ear infections by neck manipulation or "adjustment," as they call it. The infection is completely contained within a closed bony space in the skull and the cause is a living organism, a bacteria. Still, you are led to believe that allowing someone to move the child's neck for a few seconds once a day will cure the problem. Apparently allowing the child to repeat exactly the same movements at school or at play, as he nods in response to a question or she looks over her shoulder playing tag, has no effect. Sounds a little silly, and it might be if the parents weren't told that adjustments can take the place of antibiotics or even necessary surgery to drain the infection.

If you take your back problem to a chiropractor, he will almost always take an x-ray, and often the views will be in one direction only, generally from front to back, as though your spine had only two dimensions instead of three. If you saw a face-on photograph of a playing card, you'd have no idea whether it was paper-thin or an inch thick; and if you saw a photo of the same card viewed from one edge, it would resemble a thin pencil line. Either way, you'd have an inadequate notion of what a playing card looks like. The same limitations are faced by any practitioner trying to rely on a single-directional x-ray.

For completely non-scientific reasons, chiropractors often include your entire spine from head to pelvis in one x-ray. There is a small risk of unnecessary radiation, but my main objection to this practice is that the x-ray is useless. Any detail of the affected area, involving one or two levels of the spine, is lost. This type of x-ray usually comes complete with numerous wax pencil markings outlining individual vertebra or defining angles between adjacent bones. The marks have no diagnostic significance, but they certainly look impressive.

One woman, being treated by a chiropractor, brought me her low back x-ray for a second opinion. Lines drawn along the top and bottom of two vertebrae at the "source" of her trouble were connected by an arrow to the unfortunate "result," a large black spot at the upper corner of the film. She was surprised and relieved to learn the dark area was, in fact, only gas in her stomach. A discreet burp and she was "cured."

Even when they are shot thoroughly and properly, x-rays have serious limitations as a diagnostic tool. Yet chiropractors rely on x-rays extensively. Apparently some of them do not realize that the physical changes seen on the x-ray plate will not necessarily be the ones responsible for the pain you are feeling at the time. You can't x-ray pain. The wear that is causing your pain today may remain undetectable by x-ray for years. Or you may even have a painful condition that never shows up on an x-ray plate. Discs, for example, do not appear on x-rays. You can have a painful protruding disc and still have an x-ray that looks perfectly normal.

Being aware of the faith that many chiropractors have in these images, I was amused not long ago to see a chiropractor pop up on television one evening, demonstrating his use of x-rays. He was working on a patient's back, with an x-ray film conspicuously displayed on the wall nearby. As he simulated his treatment of the patient's spinal column, the chiropractor's eyes darted repeatedly between the patient and the x-ray. He gave the impression that he was closely relating the x-ray information to his manipulation of the patient's spine. What wasn't made clear was that almost nothing seen on the x-ray could be felt with the fingers. Only the backward-facing bony projections at the back of the spine are palpable. A sense of the general location of the vertebrae can be gained easily by touch alone. Did you ever drive through a busy intersection in a strange city and try to read a street map at the same time? If you don't know where you're going by then, it's too late to look. What the television audience saw that evening may have been good show business, but it was hokey medicine.

Whether they actually say so or not, many chiropractors give the impression that they can somehow place their hands on a person's spine and shift misplaced bones back into position. Anyone who harbors that concept has no realistic idea of the anatomy of the human back. I find it difficult to believe that any chiropractor who holds that view has ever attended surgery and tried to rearrange the exposed bones of the spine in an anesthetized patient. I suspect that the typical chiropractor's ideas about the interior of the human back are based on the study of skeletons conveniently stripped of their muscles, ligaments, fat, and skin. When you study the backbone that way, you gain no appreciation of the way a spine would resist manipulation.

While I agree that manipulation has its place in back treatment — for instance, in the relief of muscle spasms, or in the freeing up of stiff joints — the proponents of manipulation tend to overstate its value. I think they do this often out of a mistaken understanding of living spinal anatomy. Let me tell you about an experience I had with a person who is — or should be — as knowledgeable about the human back as any chiropractor. This person is a physiotherapist, an accredited member of the medical community.

This man — let's call him Jack — found that family doctors in his community were referring quite a number of back patients to him. For this reason, he wanted to pick up any additional skill or knowledge he could acquire on the subject of back pain. He came to me, asking for advice. I decided it would be useful for him to observe the spinal operation I was about to perform on a young woman suffering from a sequestrated disc.

Now, Jack was a man with better qualifications than the average physiotherapist. I judged him to be a person of considerable intelligence, and his credentials showed that he had trained in a first-class institution in Europe. He was a firm believer in the concept of spinal manipulation. Apparently he had accepted the idea that spines could be "adjusted" readily by movement and massage. Yet the operation he observed that day was the first back surgery he had ever seen. In other words, he had never before set eyes on the backbone of a living human being.

I made the incision. My twenty-six-year-old patient was a woman you might describe as chubby but certainly not obese. Cutting through the skin, I came first to a layer of fat about an inch (2.5 cm) thick. Beneath that, a layer of muscle — another inch. Next we encountered a second layer of muscle on the back of the spinal joints, and we stripped away a small portion of that muscle to expose the bone.

With the rearmost part of the backbone in view, we could see the roofs of those little "Monopoly houses" with the spines of the vertebrae projecting upward like tiny chimneys. We were 2 inches (5 cm), at least, beneath the surface of the patient's skin. I exposed enough bone to be able to grasp two of the spiny projections with surgical instruments. To make a point to my observing friend, I took hold of the bones and tried to move them back and forth. They budged less than a quarter of an inch (5 mm). There was no way I could "manipulate" them, even while grasping those two adjacent vertebrae with heavy forceps. With direct access to the spine in an anesthetized paralyzed patient and using strong tools, I couldn't do what that physiotherapist always thought he had been doing by pressing his fingertips against the skin of his conscious patient's back.

Another point had become obvious: manipulation could not be the precise art its proponents claim it to be. The joints in the patient's back were 2 inches (5 cm) from the surface, were identified only by slight bulges along the edge of the bony "roof," and were only half an inch (1 cm) apart. To appreciate what I'm saying here, lay two parallel rows of pennies, half a dozen in each row, on top of a table and cover them with a 2-inch (5 cm) thickness of newspaper. Now see if you can locate the second penny from the end on the left. Impossible, isn't it? Yet that's what a proponent of manipulation is claiming to do, in effect, when he purports to manipulate, say, your left facet joint at the L_4-L_5 level.

Carrying on with surgery, I penetrated the bony back of the spinal canal, worked through the cavity beyond it, and came to the disc, where I plucked out the loose fragment of disc that had been causing my patient's pain.

By now, Jack had another point to ponder: the impossibility of the so-called disc adjustment. He realized that while it's difficult enough to manipulate individual spinal joints by laying hands on the surface of the skin, it's preposterous to believe that a bulging disc can be "adjusted" by exerting direct pressure on the back. He had to ask himself how anyone's spinal discs might be affected by manual contact through that multiple barrier of skin, fat, muscle, bone, and spinal canal. The answer, of course, is that there is no way.

Put your two rows of pennies into a desk drawer, shut the drawer, and see how well you can feel them through the top of the desk. That's what a "manipulator" is doing when he feels your back and declares, "I can feel your disc is out of place."

I doubt whether one chiropractor in a hundred has seen half as much as Jack saw in that one operation. Yet many chiropractors speak glibly of realigning your L_{4-5} joint or slipping your L_{3-4} disc back into place, as though your interior body parts could be shifted around as readily as pawns on a chessboard.

Chiropractic treatment is not useless. Like any other form of skilled manipulation, it can put your spine through a useful range of movements, just as a series of bending and stretching exercises would do in a somewhat different way. And it is a fact that manipulation sometimes relieves muscle spasms, thereby reducing or eliminating pain.

And manipulation can shorten the duration of an acute attack. In other words, chiropractic has its uses for people who need what the chiropractor has to offer: the relief of some forms of acute paraspinal muscle spasm through manipulation of the neck or low back.

Certainly chiropractors go too far when they suggest that manipulation will prevent spinal problems as well as cure them. A muscle spasm, for instance, is an extreme form of tension, a tightening that occurs under physical or emotional stress. That tightness may be loosened by manipulation, but no amount of manipulation carried out when you are free of pain can prevent a spasm from happening later. The same is true of "maintaining spinal alignment" through chiropractic adjustments. The discs of your spine do not slip and the facet joints do not keep going out. Everything is already in place — there is nothing to put back. And manipulation can do nothing to prevent the natural wear that is the source of common backache. Chiropractors who suggest otherwise are either trading on the popular mystique of the back or merely revealing their own inadequate understanding of the way the back works.

In some circumstances, then, manipulation is useful, notably in the relief of acute muscle spasms. In other cases, it is useless but harmless, as in so-called maintenance therapy. I use "harmless" in reference to the physical aspects of the procedure. There is nothing "harmless" about creating unnecessary dependence in a patient with chronic backache. In very rare cases, it can be physically risky, as in a case of spinal tumor. In this instance, however, I expect the competent chiropractor to recognize that a manipulation is not advisable.

I never hesitate to recommend manipulative therapy for my patients if I believe it will be safe and useful. Although I usually send these cases to a physiotherapist with skill in manual therapy techniques, I have no difficulty in referring to a chiropractor. Both are professionals trained in a particular treatment method. The nature of their training may be different, but in the end, they have the same ability to manipulate the spine.

I do have a problem when the chiropractor finds it necessary to tell the patient that his back has a curve in it (whether it does or not) and that one leg is longer than the other (whether it is or not). It happens so often that when I see a patient who has been attending a chiropractor, I always comment that one leg seems longer. The patient is usually impressed that I noticed so quickly.

The physiotherapist generally keeps in touch with me during the treatment period. The patient's progress becomes our common concern. Many chiropractors, I am afraid, are not team players — at least not with doctors. I am optimistic, however, that there will be more cooperation in the future between chiropractors and physicians. Young chiropractors are more inclined than their elders to distinguish between back patients who can benefit from manipulation and those who require medical management. No longer is the entire profession devoted to selling chiropractic as the magic cure-all. Referrals from doctors to chiropractors and from chiropractors to doctors are becoming more frequent — a healthy sign, in my view.

By now, you may be wondering, "If the benefits of chiropractic are as limited as he says, why are chiropractors flourishing? And why do we keep hearing enthusiastic stories from people who say their chiropractor helped them after their own doctors failed?"

The answer is that chiropractors enjoy a degree of popularity out of proportion to the medical value of their art. On the basis of my own experience, discussions with thousands of back patients, and a review of the medical and chiropractic literature, you have about a sixty percent chance of relieving an acute back attack by seeing a chiropractor. That estimate, however, may make manipulation sound more effective than it is. Other factors help the chiropractor look good, especially if you go to him after a disenchanting experience with a doctor.

Here are the factors that most often work to the chiropractor's advantage.

The Last-Resort Syndrome

When your doctor fails to solve your back problem, you wonder, "Is he not a very good doctor, or am I a hopeless case? Whichever it is, what have I got to lose by trying a chiropractor?"

Well, you haven't much to lose. But once you're in that state of mind, your chiropractor can hardly lose either. After he has treated you, your back will feel better or it won't. If it feels better, the chiropractor wins full marks. He has succeeded where your doctor failed. You tell all your friends about him. If your back doesn't feel better, that's hardly the chiropractor's fault. After all, your doctor — a qualified MD — couldn't cure it either. But you don't tell your friends that you saw a doctor and a chiropractor, both of whom were no good. You tell them you have a back problem that has baffled at least two medical specialists.

Salesmanship

Let's pretend you inherited some money and are trying to choose between two investment dealers.

Mrs. A tells you: "I suppose we might, uh, find some suitable stock or bond for you, but the market is, uh, rather uncertain at the best of times. Of course, I would be willing to look into it and do whatever I could, but I must warn you that I can't guarantee . . ."

Mr. B tells you: "Look — I've made a lot of people wealthy in the past five years. Seven of my clients had to borrow bus fare to get here. Today they're millionaires. I can do the same for you. Now this is my plan . . ."

Would you believe me if I told you Mrs. A knows more about investing than Mr. B does? You wouldn't want to believe it, would you?

People with back problems have the same kind of trouble maintaining confidence in a doctor who sounds like the medical equivalent of Mrs. A. And too many doctors do. They hem and haw and neglect to communicate even half of what they know about the patient's condition or what can be done about it. To make matters worse, they mumble about arthritis and worry aloud about the possibility (extraordinarily remote) of cancer. There is nothing wrong with being thoughtful and cautious, especially in medicine, but it is self-defeating to be so non-committal and so frightening that people doubt the doctor's professional abilities.

Chiropractors don't make that mistake. When you walk into a chiropractor's office, he greets you warmly, examines you with expert aplomb, and announces: "No wonder you're having pain. Your problem is a C_{5-6} subluxation that needs to be adjusted 4 millimeters to the left. If you'd like to recline here on this table, I can look after it for you right now."

Salesmanship has another benefit: it builds the chiropractor's practice. There is no evidence whatsoever that normal healthy children require spinal adjustment, but that is just what some chiropractors recommend. Treatment should begin, they say, in the first few weeks of life and continue indefinitely. Remember the old adage, "Give me the child and I will have the man."

The reason provided most often for spinal adjustment in infants is the presence of "subluxations" inevitably caused by the trauma of normal birth. The word is Doctor. "Sub" means less than, and "luxation" is an old-fashioned term for a dislocation, a joint out of place. Subluxation, then, means the spinal joints are less than dislocated — in other words, the joints are still in place. By finding subluxations in each newborn, chiropractors are asking us to believe that, despite hundreds of millions of years of evolution, Nature has selected a method of birth that damages every newborn spine. Furthermore, spinal subluxation is a condition that cannot be identified by any known imaging technique, yet some chiropractors refer to it as "the silent killer." That's a powerful sales pitch.

Many chiropractors have spoken out against this type of approach and have suggested that chiropractic be limited to the management of acute mechanical low back pain. They have met with surprisingly strong rejection from within their own profession. Harsher critics than I have suggested that in the art of manipulation, some chiropractors are even more adept with people than with spines.

The Equality Hangup

I can explain this phenomenon by describing the experience of a colleague while he was shepherding six medical students through rounds in a hospital. In the emergency room, they came upon a woman with acute appendicitis. My friend knew what was wrong with her, but by way of teaching the art of diagnosis, he withheld that knowledge and asked each student, in turn, to examine her and give an opinion.

The first student said the patient needed her gall bladder removed. The next said she had a bowel problem. The third thought it was a stomach ulcer. And so on. Six students offered six different diagnoses — all of them wrong. Finally, my colleague enlightened them. "This woman," he announced, "has acute appendicitis. In fact, it is so acute that we are taking her to the operating room within the hour."

At that moment, the patient spoke up. "Wait a minute!" she told the doctor. "You're only one out of seven. If you guys can't agree on what's wrong with me, nobody is taking out my appendix!"

If you are a back patient who's been examined by, perhaps, four doctors who provided four different — or different-sounding — diagnoses, I can't blame you if you think the whole thing is just a guessing game, with one doctor's opinion as good as another's. If that were so, diagnosticians wouldn't need to spend time acquiring training and experience. They could diagnose you by taking a public opinion poll out on the street. But some people favor this notion of equality among experts, as though there were no degrees of experience or expertise. That is a dangerous attitude to carry with you into the office of any practitioner — doctor or chiropractor.

The Remission Factor

Sore backs have good days and bad days. For nearly ninety percent of sufferers, the acute attack is gone within six to eight weeks. If you were a person without conscience, you could use that fact to make a lot of money. You could set up a shop where you offered to make anyone's back feel better by treating it with a magic blue light. It would be just an ordinary light, of course, but your customers wouldn't know that. You'd persuade them to pay you $100 a day for an eight-week course of daily treatments. And to show how reputable you are, you offer a money-back guarantee. From the natural history alone, nine out of every ten back patients you see will be better at the end of your sessions. One person gets his money back and tells everyone how honest you are. Nine people will tell everyone they meet about your marvelous clinic and your miracle cure.

The Placebo Effect

This is a factor that works to the advantage of every practitioner at some time, and chiropractors can hardly be criticized for enjoying its benefits. But it does account partly for the credit they receive as healers. A placebo, as you probably know, is a harmless "medicine" with no medicinal value. It relieves some people of pain through the power of suggestion. Suppose you line up a hundred people, all of whom have the same chronic back pain. You give each of them a sugar pill and tell them it will relieve their pain. Statistics show that if you are convincing, more than thirty of these people will feel better. Of course, you haven't done a thing to correct the cause of their pain, but temporarily, at least, they are "cured."

A placebo does not have to be a pill. The laying on of hands can achieve the same result. Any treatment in which the practitioner touches the patient's body — such as manipulation of the spine — carries with it a powerful Placebo Effect.

Some of the most recent studies of the Placebo Effect suggest that this phenomenon may occur through the spontaneous release of endorphins, those natural opiates that are credited with the pain-relieving effect of acupuncture. If this is so, the Placebo Effect is a method of tricking a person's body into relieving pain by means of the body's own chemistry. In other words, one victim out of three, far from being the gullible "victim" of the placebo, is fortunate in unconsciously possessing the power to release body chemicals that kill pain. Which brings up an intriguing question: Can the other two-thirds of the population be trained or induced to make use of this same power?

In simpler times, long before anyone had heard of endorphins, the Placebo Effect was exploited with stunning commercial success. Just one example is the Toronto doctor who, years ago, collected a huge following by having his arthritis patients listen to a particular radio station at specified times of the day. At those times, he assured them, he was beaming soundless "healing waves" that would cure arthritis. The patient merely had to hold the affected part close to the radio speaker and — the doctor never had to say it — believe. As far as I know, the results were not recorded methodically, but it seems likely that at least a few of the faithful experienced some relief from arthritic pain.

When a new patient comes to me with acute back pain, I examine him or her and then recommend appropriate posture correction or pain-controlling exercise. Almost inevitably, the patient asks, "But aren't you going to do anything?"

And all I can say is, "But I am doing something — I'm telling you to go home and do your exercises."

That's the best prescription I can offer at that moment, but it doesn't involve pills, drugs, manipulation, heat treatment, or the laying on of healing hands. Consequently, if I want the Placebo Effect to work for me, I must be completely convincing in my assurance that the pain-control maneuvers will work, and I must be quite precise in my instructions regarding the program so that the patient feels that something effective is under way.

The Pilgrim Syndrome

The factors that work in favor of chiropractors also enhance the popularity and reputations of health spas and clinics that specialize in treating sore backs. The operators of such establishments usually manage, as well, to take advantage of what I call the Pilgrim Syndrome.

This syndrome begins in the minds of the people who say, "I don't care how much it costs — I want the best!" It may not surprise you to learn that there are doctors who are willing to cater to such wishes.

The "clinic," as its patients often come to call it, is usually located in a fairly inaccessible, if not foreign, setting. If you're off to see the Wizard, you want to look him up in Oz, not Cleveland. The clinic usually has a waiting list, implying an exclusive and selected clientele. Its principal doctors, who are often its administrators as well, have impressive qualifications, which appear to be — and probably are — recognized by the medical establishment. At the same time, these doctors make it clear that they are, by their own choosing, and by reason of their special skills and concerns, practitioners who stand apart from the main body of the profession.

The clinic's literature is clearly intended to be seductively persuasive. It is long on emotion and salesmanship and short on hard facts and medical details. Results are never described in clinical terms — only in rave notices. One establishment in California, for instance, promotes itself with a magazine-style booklet containing an article describing how its "eager and zealous" patients acquire a "new awareness of well-being, joy of living and self-renewal." The article even claims success with the "hopelessly diseased" — a feat I first thought impossible, by definition. Then I came upon a second article in which one of the "hopeless cases," a homemaker and a mother just out of her twenties, explained the secret: "miracles."

The crucial moment in her personal saga was an encounter with her visiting family, a sort of situation from which great soap opera is made:

> I'll never forget the first day I walked without the aid of my cane. My family unexpectedly decided to join me for supper. They rushed past me in the corridor, eager to catch me in the dining room. As they passed by me, I recognized them and called out to them. They turned

and stared in open-mouthed wonder, and as the wonder
turned to joy, we three embraced and tears of happiness
streamed down our faces. We knew we could make it:
Mommy was getting well!

Unfortunately for the curious reader, Mommy never
does get around to describing what was wrong with her
back or how the clinic helped her. Such details are perhaps not considered important to the readers of the clinic's promotional literature. But money is. The booklet
tells how another patient, also a woman, "successfully
rehabilitated" in only sixty-three days after four years in
bed with a bad back, ran up a bill of $38,000. The clinic
didn't get all of that amount; part of it was for "prior
expense" and part of it for "related settlements" (whatever those two items mean), and the rest (amount unspeci-
fied) was for "our program charge."

Far from seeing this sum as exorbitant — and who can
say she didn't get full value for the money? — the administrators of the clinic calculate that without their treatment the woman's medical insurance company would
have paid out $328,000 "to support this lady's anticipat-
ed lifetime need for drugs, medical care, food, shelter,
and clothing." By a process of unassailable mathematics,
they calculate that the woman's $38,000 bill thus repre-
sented a saving to the insurance company of a tidy
$290,000. In fact, in treating sixty patients annually and
saving them an average of $200,000 apiece, this
California clinic estimates that it is saving patients or
their insurance companies $12 million a year.

Any doctor, especially a back doctor, may encounter
the Pilgrim Syndrome without having encouraged it.
This has happened to me, even though I have not yet
issued bulletins on how many millions I am saving the
insurance industry every year. My most memorable pilgrim was a middle-aged woman — from California, ironically — who had decided that a trek to Toronto would
be her salvation. She was in such bad shape she felt she
needed an ambulance to bring her from the airport. I

quickly realized that her mild Pattern One pain was not the real problem. She had developed a complete lifestyle built around her back pain, with which she ruled her family and dominated her husband. Throughout her stay in Toronto, our team administered copious amounts of positive psychology, motivation, knowledge, active physiotherapy, and sympathetic listening.

In three weeks, she was up and about and ready to go home. As she walked happily out of our facility, without the use of her cane, she couldn't find words glowing enough to express her gratitude. Apparently this woman had experienced the same sort of "awareness of well-being" and "self-renewal" advertised by that clinic in her home state — but at one-tenth the cost. Rather than the $38,000 incurred by the woman who had been "successfully rehabilitated" in sixty-three days, our patient managed her twenty-one day recovery for something less than $4,000, including treatment, accommodation, and airfare.

The moral of this story? Buyer beware. But beyond that maxim, remember that dependence on less conventional or "alternative" medicine is simply unnecessary. The power to control and relieve your back pain lies with you.

8 Step Into My Examining Room

I hope some readers of this book will find that they can apply my advice with such rewarding results that they will never have to see a doctor about their backs.

There are bound to be many more, however, who for various reasons will have their back problems diagnosed professionally. In case you become one of them, you ought to have some idea of what to expect. You will be doing both your doctor and yourself a favor if you go prepared to answer his questions and undergo an examination without any qualms about the things he will do to you.

Every doctor has his or her own style and favorite techniques, but the description here of my procedure is fairly typical of what you can expect when you see your own doctor.

If you come to me complaining of pain in your lower back, I begin with a series of questions about your medical history and personal habits. Although you may find it hard to believe, this direct low-tech approach is the most important and useful stage of your examination. I begin by asking where your pain is worse, in the back or the leg. (For patients with neck symptoms, I ask them to choose between their neck and arm.) Almost everyone has pain in both areas, but one area usually predominates, and that allows me to choose between Patterns One and Two, and Patterns Three and Four. Next, I obtain the details of your current attack — the speed of onset and duration, for example. I want to know if your pain is constant or intermittent: does it come and go? When first asked, most people reply they have constant pain. But if they can be completely objective, they almost always recall brief moments during the day when the pain disappears. Perhaps you have a certain position or can twist in just the right way to make the pain stop. Understanding the reason for those fleeting intervals of relief may be the key to your success. I will question you about any previous attacks. What things make the pain worse? What things seem to make it better? I need to understand how your pain affects your life, what it prevents you from doing.

I also ask about your general health and personal background: past illnesses; surgery, if any; patterns of illness in your family; details about your job, your work habits, your recreational pursuits.

You will be helping us both if you answer my questions not just frankly but precisely too. It's not enough, for instance, merely to say that you have pain in your back and legs. I'm going to ask you to be more specific. I want to know exactly where — only in your thigh or right down into your toes? And is there numbness or tingling, or a sensation of burning or cold?

Once I've heard your history, I have an idea about the source of your pain. Now I test my theory with the physical examination. I ask you to strip down to your underwear and slip into an examining gown that opens at the back. The examination will consist of a standard sequence of observations and tests, to be done while you are standing, sitting, kneeling, bending, and lying in various positions. The whole examination can take no more than five minutes.

If you tried the self-diagnosis set out in Chapter Four, you will recognize many of the tests I describe here. To begin, I ask you to stand up and show me how you can bend your upper body forward and backward. I assess the rhythm of your movement and, more importantly, question you about the effect repeated movement has on your typical pain. Often I suggest a pain scale from zero, no pain, to ten, the most severe the pain ever gets, to help you describe what you feel. Pain that increases as you continue bending forward indicates Pattern One. Pain aggravated with repeated backward bending is Pattern Two. Pain that is present only when you are bent all the way in one direction or the other, but that disappears as soon as you stand straight again, is likely the result of nothing more than tight tissue.

It's always surprising for people to learn that, in most cases, these few movements are the only portions of the examination that yield positive information. The remaining tests are designed to rule out the presence of direct pressure on a nerve root, Pattern Three or Four. These patterns, as you know, account for about ten percent of back pain cases, but dismissing them consumes most of the time spent in physical testing.

While you are still standing, I ask you to rise up on your toes ten times on both feet at once, then ten times, in turn, on each foot separately. Here, I am looking for any sign that a pinched nerve might have made one calf weaker than the other.

I ask you next to kneel on a chair while I test your ankle reflexes by tapping your Achilles' tendons. Differences in your reflexes from one ankle to another will also suggest the possibility of a damaged nerve.

Now I ask you to sit on a chair with your feet flat on the floor. Squatting in front of you, I press down firmly with my hand on the top of each foot in turn to see how well you can sustain elevation of your forefoot against my downward pressure. Again, I am looking for clues to Pattern Three or Pattern Four.

Incidentally, this is a test where it is impossible to fake weakness. I am not suggesting that you have come into my office pretending to have back pain that isn't there. Very few people do that. But quite a number of patients are fearful that certain limitations are so faint or subtle that they will be overlooked during the examination. And so they exaggerate these conditions, to make sure the doctor will take due note of them. Let me advise you against this inclination, because it can backfire. A doctor who realizes you are exaggerating your condition may decide that you are a complete fake. If that happens, he may ignore genuine signs of trouble.

In any case, you can't deceive me with the foot-raising test I just described. I am looking for muscular weakness. If your foot is truly weak, it will sink to the floor smoothly under my downward pressure. If it is normal, you will find it impossible to simulate that smooth downward motion. Either you let go suddenly, or else your foot will descend in a series of little "cogwheel" steps, which any competent examiner can detect. A good back examination is designed to cross-check certain findings. People who are trying to provide false information may be able to fake one test, but they will be caught out by another that should match but doesn't.

Next I have you stand facing the examining table, bending forward to rest your forearms on the bed. Now I feel with my fingertips the muscles of your back and the bumps along your spine. I feel for deformities, abnormal curvatures, and muscle spasm. Even though I am gentle, you may find it necessary to let me know, in words or with gasps or flinches, whenever I come to a tender spot. Those tender places, by the way, are not necessarily the prime sources of your pain. It is altogether likely that they are points of "referred" pain — that is, pain radiated from some other location.

I mentioned the concept of referred pain during my anatomy lesson. It is an effect everyone recognizes. We are aware that the pain of a heart attack is often felt most acutely in the left arm. That's because the nerves that supply the heart travel on to supply the arm. Once pain from the heart enters the system, the brain has no way to determine exactly where it originated and so it senses pain anywhere the nerves travel. The damage is in the heart; the pain is in the arm. For the same reason, the exact location of the sore spots around your spine is of little importance.

In your next position, you are seated on the edge of the examining table as I test your knee reflexes. Here again I am looking for differences between one leg and the other.

Now it's time for you to lie on the table, face up, as I test your hips — first by having you draw your knees up to your chest, then by turning your feet gently outward, to rotate your hip joints. If either test causes your typical pain, I'll look further for hip problems.

Chances are we will go on to the next tests, those for an irritated nerve. While you remain face up on the table, I lift your leg with the knee held straight to see whether this causes a recurrence of your typical leg pain, somewhere from the back of your thigh down to your foot. I may also press behind your knee at the point where the sciatic nerve passes close to the bone. If the nerve is irritated, the extra pressure of my thumb will further increase the typical pain up or down your leg.

I also check for normal nerve function by lightly pricking your legs and feet with a pin and by testing power in muscles I haven't tested so far.

Now I check to see whether your back pain might be originating from some other part of your body, by gently pressing on your kidneys and abdomen and by checking the pulses in your legs.

I make sure that you are not suffering from damage to your spinal cord by stroking the soles of your feet with the pointed handle of my reflex hammer. If your spinal cord is free of problems, your normal reflex will make your toes curl.

I may do further muscle-power tests while you lie first on one side and then on the other.

In the last position of my examination sequence, you are lying face down on the table as I lift your legs backward one at a time. If the nerve that runs from your back into the front of your leg is irritated, you will feel well-recognized pain in the front of your thigh.

Next, I test the power of your buttock muscles — by pressing on your buttocks while you alternately tense and relax them. Weakness on one side or the other is an indication that you might have Pattern Three or Four problems. This is another test where it's difficult for a patient to fake the result. That means it's useful in helping me decide whether a patient is exaggerating the symptoms. It is very difficult to tighten just one of your buttocks at a time, as you can discover for yourself.

Using light pinpricks or a wisp of cotton, I test sensation in the narrow space between your upper buttocks. A complete loss of sensation here indicates serious nerve damage. This finding, if combined with an abnormality revealed during a rectal examination, would prompt me to immediate action. There is a very serious and extremely rare variation of Pattern Three that requires emergency surgery. This is such a rare condition that in the course of examining tens of thousands of back patients, I have seen fewer than a dozen of these cases. It is the only exception to the general rule that low back pain can be treated with posture correction and exercise for several weeks or longer before giving any thought to additional medical management. If there is a loss of sensation between the buttocks and typical leg pain in both legs produced by lifting either leg alone, I am worried about a very large disc protrusion pressing on a number of nerves that control bowel and bladder function. A disc bulge of this type, which the doctor calls a central disc herniation, produces a serious condition known as acute cauda equina syndrome.

Depending on what I've found so far, I may do a rectal examination. With a rectal, I'll check the muscle tone, or resiliency, and the constriction reflex of the anal sphincter as further signs of acute damage to the cauda equina. As I have already stressed, this is an extremely rare condition, and I bring it up only because it offers one reason for a rectal examination, which otherwise may not be necessary in the course of a standard examination of your back. If you are a man, this examination includes feeling the prostate gland, which is one location that is always checked for the possibility of cancer.

That would complete your first visit, and chances are I could diagnose your problem as one of the four patterns of common back pain.

At this point, you may be wondering why I haven't

ordered x-rays, blood samples, or other tests. Well, I could do so, of course, but they would have much less value in a case of common backache than finding out whether you respond to simple treatment — posture correction, gentle stretching, and modification of your daily routine. Whether you are just recovering from an acute attack or suffering from chronic back pain, I want to see whether you improve with this conservative treatment.

If you haven't improved in a few weeks, there would still be plenty of time to explore the possibility of some other cause, such as disease or structural abnormality. You might consider this a rather casual attitude on my part, but it's not. The rarer causes that attack suddenly and develop quickly, such as central disc herniation, always include telltale symptoms that I would detect on your first visit. The rare conditions that can't be detected so readily take months to develop. A few weeks' delay would make no difference to your chances of recovery.

The likeliest outcome of that conservative treatment is that your back will show marked improvement. I have found that one-third of the patients with chronic backache who return to me in two months are completely pain-free. Another one-third of them are showing enough improvement that we know the treatment is working well; their recovery will just take a little longer. The other third show no improvement. By questioning this group, however, I have discovered that two out of three of these people have failed to improve because they have ignored the routine I've set out for them.

That leaves only about ten percent of my chronic patients with unexplained backache. These are the people who should have some additional diagnostic work done, in case their back pain is not the result of normal wear or in the event that we need to prepare for surgery.

Now that you realize that the great majority of people who come to me are helped by simple, conservative treatment, I'm sure you can see why I don't believe in spending time and money on x-rays or tests for every patient who walks into my office.

Generally speaking, the x-rays and other additional tests used in diagnosing back problems can accomplish only two things:

1. They can help pinpoint the location of trouble by showing where abnormal conditions exist.
2. They can help rule out generalized disease by showing that the patient does not have the specific findings that such a disease would cause.

Pinpointing the exact location of, say, a worn facet joint is a wasteful exercise for anyone who is going to treat the whole back with posture control and exercise. It couldn't matter less whether the trouble is at L_{4-5} or L_5-S_1, joints separated by less than the width of a finger.

And as for the function of ruling out disease or structural abnormality, proper conservative care and treatment will accomplish that too — without the risk, pain, expense, or use of professional time that some medical tests entail.

Please do not misunderstand what I am saying here. I am not implying for a moment that I consider diagnostic tests unnecessary or valueless; far from it. In fact, I use them frequently. I am saying that most patients can do without them because their backs get better so rapidly that further investigation is unnecessary.

In case you are a back patient who requires x-ray or additional testing, let me offer you a brief description and a personal opinion of each examination.

Plain X-Rays

These are the x-rays most of us have had at some time — at the dentist or during a routine check for chest disease. The x-ray is a useful tool, but it has severe limitations. Many patients, I know, think of the x-ray as a sort of medical photograph. I only wish it were that good. If I take an x-ray of your back, the film does not show a photo of your spine; it shows just a shadow cast by the bones of your back and by the other parts of your body as the rays pass through — or fail to pass through — these structures.

Furthermore, an x-ray is a photographic negative. This means that the more it is exposed to light, the darker the film becomes. This can be confusing in itself, as you will recall from what you saw the last time you looked at the negative of a favorite snapshot. The bones of your spine absorb the x-ray beam and therefore appear white on the x-ray plate. The other parts, such as muscles and internal organs, allow much of the beam to pass through, producing darker areas on the film. Reading an x-ray is like trying to "read" the intricate pattern on a painted lampshade by looking only at the shadows it casts on a nearby wall — and doing the whole thing in reverse. A single x-ray of your spine can't reveal nearly enough. Views from several angles or centered at various levels are necessary.

While an x-ray shows bone and dense muscle, other tissue appears only faintly. It doesn't show nerves or discs, except as dark spaces beside the whiteness of bones, and their shape is implied rather than visible. An x-ray will show neither a physical change in a muscle nor a muscle spasm. And, of course, it cannot show pain.

It will show a fracture. It can show an advanced case of wear. It can show the little bony projections we call bone spurs or, more properly, osteophytes. It will show a case of scoliosis, which is abnormal sideways curvature of the spine. It can show the bony destruction caused by cancer, although almost half of the bone mass must be gone before a plain x-ray can detect any change. It will show a vertebra that has slipped out of line (spondylolisthesis) or a vertebra with a defect in the bone bridge between the facet joints (spondylolysis) or an alteration that has taken place in the normal segmentation of the lumbar and sacral regions.

I remember hearing my father say he had an extra bone in his back. When I saw his x-rays I realized that what he had is technically called lumbarization. Translated from Doctor, it means that one of the five normally fused sacral vertebrae fails to join with the rest and is left as a movable bone in the lumbar region, separated from the sacrum by a fully formed disc. In effect, people with lumbarization have six lumbar vertebrae instead of the customary five, but only four sacral vertebrae instead of five. The total number of vertebrae in the spine is consistent; they are just divided differently. Some people have the opposite variation — six sacral vertebrae and four lumbar vertebrae (sacralization). A few doctors suspect that these unusual forms of segmentation may cause back pain, but this suspicion has never been confirmed.

An x-ray can show signs of soft tissue swelling if this poorly seen structure happens to be adjacent to an empty space that absorbs no x-ray. It can show certain patterns indicating such diseases as rheumatoid arthritis or ankylosing spondylitis. It would be unusual, however, to discover these diseases by x-ray alone, since their symptoms should be obvious during a routine physical examination.

An x-ray can be much more useful if it has some basis for comparison. The x-ray you have taken next week will tell your doctor a lot more if he can compare it with the same view taken a few years earlier. That is one reason why it is not a good idea for someone with back trouble to switch doctors without a referral. Sometimes when I ask new patients about old x-rays, they say, "My other doctor has some, but I'd rather you didn't call him." When that happens, my hands are tied. It may take a little courage on your part to tell a doctor you're leaving him, but you won't be the first. In any medical practice, patients come and go. If you don't make that little exit speech so your x-rays and records can be passed along, you are depriving your new doctor — and yourself — of an important advantage.

Blood Tests

From a small sample of your blood, a medical laboratory can tell me a lot about the health of your back.

A hemoglobin test will tell me about the condition of your bone marrow, where your red blood cells are made, and about the iron storage available throughout your body. A low hemoglobin can mean a lot of things, but it may reflect a problem in normal bone marrow function and that could be related to back pain.

A count and analysis of white blood cells can indicate infection or problems with the immune system. Bone infection, or osteomyelitis, is a rare cause of acute back pain.

A sedimentation rate — the speed with which your red blood cells settle in a glass tube — is an old-fashioned but useful test for ruling out the possibility of widespread disease as the cause of your back pain. The test is very non-specific, which means it is altered by a large number of unrelated conditions. Still, it is a surprisingly useful means of detecting some systemic illnesses.

Rheumatoid factor and *anti-nuclear antibodies* are two tests to detect rheumatoid disease or other similar illnesses. These diseases belong to a group called sero-positive diseases, meaning that the diagnosis often can be made by examining the serum, part of the blood. But these tests are not infallible, and no laboratory test, however accurate, can be expected to replace what a doctor learns from a patient's history and physical examination.

Blood calcium, phosphorus, and various enzymes. When rapid changes occur in the structure of the bone, calcium, phosphorus, and certain enzymes appear in the blood in increased amounts. They reflect the bones' reaction to several types of bone-forming or bone-destroying cancers and a variety of diseases that affect bone. Normal levels of these minerals and complex proteins will help rule out the possibility of cancer or generalized disease as a cause of back pain.

Urine Tests

Some systemic illnesses and some types of cancer can also be detected by examining the urine.

Electromyography and Nerve-Conduction Studies

Although these are two separate tests, they are often carried out together because they are done with the same equipment. Electromyography (EMG) is a means of studying the reaction of a muscle when it is stimulated by a nerve. A nerve-conduction study is the examination of a specific nerve's ability to conduct impulses.

Suppose, for example, that you have back pain and have lost the ability to lift your toes while your foot is flat on the floor. The culprit may be the muscle or the sciatic nerve or the nerve root that governs that foot action. The first possibility can be ruled out by the EMG, and the other two by a nerve-conduction study.

To conduct these tests, the examiner will insert extremely fine needles at several points along the length of your leg. The test is uncomfortable but not painful. The needles are wired to an instrument that can show whether your muscular contraction and nerve impulses are normal. If they are, the doctor can conclude — by simple deduction — that the damage is located higher up, at the nerve root.

Newer techniques using surface electrodes instead of needles are being developed and may widen the application of these procedures.

Few patients with common backache require these tests. They are of no use in Pattern One or Pattern Two because these patterns have no direct interference with nerve function. The picture in Pattern Three can be identified just as clearly from the history and physical examination. Tests in Pattern Four are routinely normal because the patient is at rest and, in Pattern Four, nerve problems occur only with exercise.

Somatosensory-Evoked Potentials

SSEP for short or SEP (even shorter) is a new technique that measures the effect on certain areas in the brain of stimulating the spinal cord or even an individual nerve. It is used during surgery to warn the surgeon of impending neural damage, or to indicate when a nerve root has been adequately decompressed. It is not yet in wide use; it is expensive and requires a team of highly trained technicians. But one exciting possibility is that it may form the basis of a means to actually measure pain.

Bone Scanning

Certain changes in the bones of your spine can be located by injecting a harmless radioactive material into your bloodstream. Within a couple of hours the material is incorporated into your bones. Its radiation, picked up by a device comparable to a Geiger counter, can be displayed on a screen or recorded as a "picture" similar to an x-ray. In a location where there is rapid bone turnover, such as in a healing fracture, the repair of a worn joint, or a bone-forming cancer, the increased amount of uptake and radioactivity is indicated by a dense black area or "hot spot" on the film. The test is safe and painless and the radioactive material disappears rapidly.

Thermography

This test was devised to pinpoint trouble spots by detecting altered circulation. It is based on the theory that where there is inflammation, there will be extra heat on the surface of the skin, created by an increased concentration of blood. Also, it is a fact that your nerves control the diameter of your blood vessels; therefore, if you have something wrong with a nerve, the size of the blood vessels may be altered and the flow of blood will be affected.

Personally, I believe this test has no place in the diagnosis of back pain. There is no proven correlation between the thermogram picture and either the pattern or the physical source of the pain.

Ultrasound

Ultrasound is generating a great deal of enthusiasm among doctors in other specialties, and for good reason. But as a tool for diagnosing back problems, it is just beyond the experimental stage. It is a noble attempt to gather as much information as possible about your spine without invading your body or subjecting it to excessive radiation in the process. A machine bounces high-frequency sound waves harmlessly off the structures in your back, and the resulting waves create a rather imprecise "picture" of your spine. X-rays are hard enough to interpret, but ultrasound results are even more difficult. Still, the techniques are continuing to be refined, and as the quality of the image improves, the role of ultrasound may grow.

Tomography

Although rarely used anymore, tomography of the spine marked an important step in the evolution of spinal x-rays. It is also the technique upon which the CT scan is based. Tomography produces a series of x-ray pictures, each taken at a slightly different depth in your body. Perhaps I can describe this process more clearly by using a child's birthday cake as an example of an x-ray subject. Suppose you made a traditional birthday cake and dropped several dozen coins into it at random. If you x-rayed the cake to locate the coins, you'd see only a confusing jumble of overlapping shapes, with no indication whether a given coin was close to the surface or deep inside. A more reliable way of getting this information would be to cut a series of thin, parallel slices of cake, to see whether they contained any coins. Of course, we can't slice up your body or your spine that way, but the tomograph does that for us in pictures. It produces a dozen or so x-rays, each one a cut deeper than the last. Since we know the depth at which each cut was made, we can accurately identify the location of the objects we see in each picture. By studying the whole series of images, we can construct in our minds a composite picture of what your spine must look like.

The Myelogram

Like the tomogram, in many centers myelography is disappearing from the investigation of spinal problems, replaced by the CT scan or the magnetic resonance image. Still, it remains the standard against which all other techniques to show the nerves are measured. The myelogram uses an x-ray machine in conjunction with a colorless liquid that is radiopaque — that is, impervious to x-rays.

The test begins with the injection of the fluid into the patient's dural sac, which is the sheath surrounding the spinal cord and the nerve roots. The patient lies on a tilting table, and as x-rays are shot, he is tilted back and forth so that the injected material flows slowly up and down his spine as it fills the space surrounding each nerve. The fluid appears white on the x-rays, while the indentations or outright obstructions from protruding discs show up as dark blotches. The myelogram does not show the discs. It outlines the defect a disc produces as it presses against the nerve sac.

A myelogram is not infallible. It may show an indentation from a bulging disc that is not, in fact, the cause of your pain. Or the bulging disc that is responsible may remain undetected on the myelogram because it is pushing against the nerve in a portion of the dural sac that contains none of the test fluid. The myelogram is always normal in Patterns One and Two, where no nerve pressure occurs.

The myelogram must be used with caution. Some people suffer headaches after a myelogram, but the discomfort usually disappears within twenty-four hours if the patient rests flat in bed. The headaches may last longer and will sometimes carry a suggestive effect that lasts indefinitely. Rightly or wrongly, a few patients insist that their backs became worse after a myelogram. Even if that's not true, it's a problem for any patient who believes it.

I believe strongly that myelography should not used as a routine diagnostic tool. Except in instances where the patient's condition defies diagnosis by less invasive forms of observation and testing, a myelogram should be avoided. It still has a place in the precise localization of root compression before surgery in a patient with Pattern Three or Four leg-dominant pain. As a general rule, if you are not willing to have surgery, you should not have a myelogram.

The Discogram

This is another technique involving injection of a liquid opaque to x-rays. In this case, however, the material is injected directly into the disc and the test is graded by the patient's pain response, not by the x-ray picture. In a normal disc, the injected fluid, unable to escape, shows on x-ray as an almond-shaped or dumbbell-shaped blob inside the disc, centered between the two adjacent vertebrae. If the disc is ruptured or badly worn, the injected fluid leaks out quickly and disappears.

It's a painful test. No anesthetic is used, and the conclusions drawn depend primarily (I think it should be almost exclusively) on the test's ability to reproduce precisely the patient's typical pain. To me, an equivocal answer is not proof enough that we have identified the source of pain. As well, it is a difficult test to administer; the needle must be inserted in precisely the right location within the disc and the patient must be asked exactly the right questions. To add to the widespread distrust of this test, the x-ray picture may show a damaged disc that causes no pain or a normal disc that reproduces the symptoms.

Nerve-Root Injection

The purpose of this test is to determine which nerve root is to blame for an area of leg pain. A radiopaque liquid and a local anesthetic are mixed together and injected around the suspected root. The opaque fluid shows up on a fluoroscope, confirming that the correct nerve root has been injected. The anesthetic, of course, removes all feeling from that branch. If the pain ceases, the doctor knows he has located the trouble spot — *more or less*.

The problem is that adjacent nerve roots overlap in function. Instead of pinpointing the nerve root where the pain is originating, the test may throw suspicion upon an "innocent" neighbor that is merely relaying the pain message.

Facet Injection

Working on the same principle as the nerve-root injection and with the same mixture of fluids, this test helps determine which joint is to blame for facet pain. In my opinion, it's more accurate than a nerve-root injection, although the same overlap can occur, raising the same questions as to where the pain signals actually originated. Even pinpointing the origin of the pain, however, doesn't solve the problem of what to do next. Unless the need for surgery is obvious — and it seldom is — conservative management may be the most sensible treatment. In that case, it doesn't really matter which particular facet joint is causing the pain, and the test shouldn't be done.

Some doctors add steroids to the injection to try to reduce inflammation within the joint and relieve symptoms. It seems like a fine idea, but there is no evidence that it has any lasting effect.

The CT Scanner

Computerized tomography, or to use the full name, computerized axial tomography, is a fancy x-ray. But calling it that is like saying the space shuttle is a complicated flying machine.

By comparison, the output of the CT scanner makes tomography looks like drawings on some caveman's wall. The tomogram produces its dozen or so serial x-rays of the bone structure of the back, but leaves their interpretation entirely to a human expert. The CT scanner combines its own multiple exposures into pictures with astounding clarity and easy-to-read detail.

The CT scanner's strength lies partly in the way its computer can "read" the subtle differences it sees between one x-ray and the next — differences no human eye could ever detect. Having read these differences, the CT then accentuates them, all in proportion to their original intensity, so that they can be seen at a glance. In practical terms, this means that the CT, far from being limited to showing bony structures, can portray soft tissue. It can actually take pictures of the membranes surrounding the nerve; it can even show the internal structure of the spinal cord itself.

The CT's computer can also work by inference to "show" views that even it has never seen. For instance, it can show a side view that would be impossible to x-ray. It does this by taking many views of a frontal exposure, each at a slightly different depth. By detecting and "remembering" the subtle differences it has seen from one depth to the next, the CT can portray — by deductive memory — precisely what a side view must look like. It can even reconstruct the spine in three dimensions.

The CT scan does have limitations. For this reason, it is sometimes combined with a myelogram. The contrast material fills the sac around the nerve roots as in any myelogram. But now the CT does more than just display the filling defect; it actually shows the disc that is applying the pressure. That's something the myelogram alone can't do. CT myelography takes us a long way towards the ideal image, but it still falls short. And that's where MRI comes in.

Magnetic Resonance Imaging

MRI can get the views the CT and even the myelogram CT can't manage.

The MRI operates by subjecting your body to an intense magnetic field, many thousands of times stronger than the earth's magnetic pull. As you lie in a narrow space within the machine, your body's molecules line up, just like the iron filings around a bar magnet in that old experiment from public school. When the situation is stable, you are subjected to a powerful radio signal that briefly pushes the molecules out of alignment, much like the effect of tapping a spinning top: it wobbles, then returns to its steady vertical position. As they realign themselves, all of your molecules emit weak electrical signals. A computer, tuned to the frequency of hydrogen (chosen because it is plentiful in the body and broadcasts a clear message) records each discharge, noting the strength and location, and then generates a picture. The mathematics are mind-numbing, but the result is a picture of your body outlined in hydrogen. (Since two hydrogen and one oxygen make H_2O, it's actually drawn with water.) The result looks like an x-ray, but it's really a computer-generated picture, like the "pictures" of Jupiter sent to earth by computer from Voyager II.

The MRI can show us the whole body, anywhere there is water. Because of their low water content, bones appear black while discs, muscles and nerves are white. The lack of moisture in the bones is a drawback; the bone images are not as clear as a high-resolution CT. But for the other tissues, the MRI is unequaled. We can locate changes in the bone marrow and pinpoint cancers before they have a chance to spread. We can examine disc protrusions so small they are hard to see at surgery. We can determine the degree of water loss in a disc and watch the splitting of its shell.

We can find so many possible causes for common backache that we can't decide which ones to treat. The MRI has given us answers to questions we haven't even asked. For patients suffering from rare causes of non-mechanical back pain or as a prelude to necessary surgery, magnetic imaging is invaluable. But even the MRI can't see pain, and it doesn't provide the means of controlling common backache. If it's your back, that's still up to you.

9 *Poultices, Pulleys, and Pills*

Just as there is no scarcity of practitioners willing to treat your back pain, there is no shortage of backache remedies to choose from — old and new, simple and sophisticated, home-brewed and professionally prescribed. You could almost say that in addition to their bulging discs, worn facets, and pinched nerves, the victims of common backache can't seek relief without suffering from a fourth complaint: overchoice.

Hot packs or ice? Traction or massage? Injections or surgery? Everybody you talk to has a different remedy and, usually, a personal testimonial to go with it. How do you sort it all out? First, you have to decide whether you want to treat the cause or simply relieve the pain. No doubt you would like to do both. But when the pain is at its peak, you would settle gratefully for relief alone. And there's nothing the matter with that. After all, it will give you a chance to achieve some comfort and rest while your back goes about the tedious but welcome process of healing itself.

You do want to make sure, however, that the interim remedies you use are safe — free of serious side effects and not injurious. A sound rule to remember is: No pain control remedy should make you feel worse. And the converse is true: If it feels good, do it.

It's commendable to apply the power of positive thinking to your personal recovery program, but you should never deceive yourself about the value of any remedy. It pays to know, as precisely as you can, how a given therapy is supposed to work, what it can be expected to do for your back, and whether its beneficial effects are likely to last. And in assessing any back treatment, remember that back pain naturally tends to come and go, and that this may occur coincidentally with the application of your therapy, giving you a false impression of its effectiveness. You should be wary, meanwhile, of becoming dependent on short-term measures such as medication or a back brace. These are poor substitutes for a program of proper, long-term back care.

In plotting a course for your long-term recovery, you should begin by understanding the purpose and worth of each short-term pain control technique. Some are medically proven; others are based on unproven theories that may or may not be valid. Still others produce limited or erratic results. And there are a few treatments that are patently phony.

The Back Brace

A back brace can be good for you. The trouble is, people often misunderstand why. They assume, erroneously, that a brace protects the discs and helps strengthen your spine. A brace does limit excessive back movement and it is there as a reminder every time you lift or twist in an unusual position. There is a little evidence to suggest that the brace adds support for your belly muscles, although, surprisingly, this is probably not a particularly important function. But these are temporary benefits, and substituting a brace for weak muscles is not a wise long-term plan. The danger is that a brace will become a crutch. If you rely on it indefinitely, your trunk muscles will never grow strong. You are far better off to get started on an exercise program to strengthen those muscles, and meanwhile use a brace only on occasions when you cannot get along without it.

If I recommend a brace at all, I specify that it is one that can be worn outside your clothes and be loosened easily when not required. I also stress that the use of a brace must be part of a total back care program, including proper lifting techniques, regular exercise, and sensible changes in your daily routine.

Mattresses and Car Seats

People with back trouble worry a lot about mattresses. In most cases, their worries are unfounded. If you sleep on a good, firm mattress supported on a standard box spring, you are providing your back with most of the help it needs each night. There is no advantage or virtue in sleeping on a hard, uncomfortable surface — unless you enjoy it. The extravagant claims made for waterbeds or special orthopedic mattresses are based on the simple fact that they supply contoured support for the back to maintain it in a neutral position. Studies have shown that you move less often when you sleep on a waterbed. If staying in one position, ideally a comfortable one, for a longer time makes you feel good, you'll love your waterbed.

Forget the old idea of a rigid board under the mattress. That idea had merit at one time. But those were the days when beds consisted of link springs and stuffed mattresses that sagged like a swaybacked horse on its way to the glue factory. A bed like that provided virtually no support for your spine, and in that situation a rigid board made sense. If your mattress feels comfortable when your back is pain-free, it's giving you all the support you need.

No matter what sort of mattress you use, you'll probably be more comfortable during times of back pain if you lie on your back with a fat pillow under your knees, or on your side with your knees bent and a pillow between your thighs. A rolled towel around your waist often helps. I'll talk more about sleep positions in Chapter 13.

There is no magic formula for the ideal car seat, either. But one basic principle is important: keep your knees higher than your hips to hold the proper neutral curve in your low back. That means positioning your car seat as close as possible to the steering wheel — within the bounds of safety and comfort, of course. This position causes you to bend your legs and reduce the strain on your back. For comfort and good visibility, you may want to sit on a wedge-shaped cushion or place a rolled pillow in the small of your back. But let common sense prevail; whatever arrangement reduces your back pain is the right arrangement for you.

Traction

Traction is one form of treatment that has more effect on the neck than on the low back. Because it is a smaller structure, the neck can stretch and increase the space for the spinal nerves within their exit canals. For this reason, traction can be excellent therapy for Pattern Three neck and arm-dominant pain, the result of an acutely pinched nerve. To be most effective, traction should be applied frequently. For extremely painful cases, 7 to 10 pounds (3 to 4.5 kg) of pull on the head applied for several minutes every hour may help. The position of the neck is very important. Traction in one position, with the neck bent slightly forward, for example, may reduce the pain, whereas traction with the neck bent backward may not. You need to experiment using a simple traction system: a head halter, a rope, a pulley, and a weight bag.

Like any temporary treatment intended to reduce your pain without changing the underlying condition, traction should improve your symptoms, and it should do so within the first few treatments. Avoid traction if it makes your typical arm pain worse.

Traction is seldom an effective remedy for people with low back pain. The size of the trunk, the bulk of the back muscles, and even the shape of the vertebrae makes stretching of the lumbar spine extremely difficult. Some people spend a lot of money on traction devices or attend clinics for regular traction treatments that purport to reduce a disc bulge or improve the alignment of the bones in their low back. Then they lie in bed, letting the apparatus do its thing. As far as I can see, the only beneficial aspect to this treatment is that it induces you to lie down. You could throw away the weights, ropes, and pulleys and achieve just as much simply by lying in bed and allowing your back pain to subside temporarily by itself.

One variation of this treatment is called gravity traction. It uses an apparatus that leaves you hanging vertically, suspended from the chest area, in a sort of Jolly Jumper for grown-ups. Thus, in contrast with traditional, in-bed traction, which provides 40 or 50 pounds (18 to 23 kg) of pull at the most, gravity traction subjects your spine to the pull exerted by the weight of your entire lower body. There are some types of gravity traction that leave you hanging upside-down, like a bat in a cave. You can hang by your ankles or be strapped into an inverted chair.

If you are convinced that one of these latest incarnations of the medieval rack is good for the spine, let me make a suggestion: with a little more effort, but no expense whatever, you can achieve the same effect by suspending yourself by your arms, trapeze-artist style, from any convenient fixture in your house. A door frame or an overhead water pipe in your basement might do.

Try it. You might like it. But remember, traction for the low back is just one more way of relieving a muscle spasm that might go away as rapidly with a shift in posture or a gentle stretching exercise.

Counter-Irritants

Some of the most familiar home remedies are based on the principle of altering your body's perception of pain. This is done by introducing a counter-irritant that causes some new form of pain. No one knows exactly how counter-irritants work. They may release endorphins that relieve pain, or they may jam pain signals so that the body cannot register them fully and accurately.

Hot poultices and *ice packs* are probably the oldest, as well as the commonest, counter-irritants known to man.

Liniments, especially those that feel hot on the skin, are another form of counter-irritant. But don't believe the label on the liniment bottle if it claims that the product will provide "penetrating heat" that gets "deep down into the sore area."

That doesn't happen. Your skin is such an effective insulator that it blocks off any heat or cold that you might apply to your back. Certainly no liniment gets as far down as a disc or facet joint and, even if it did, there's no reason to believe that the heat or irritation would have any physical effect on the sore spots.

Massage, with or without liniment, may function as a counter-irritant. Or it may help loosen up muscles that have gone into spasm. In cases where a muscle spasm happens to be causing most of the pain, massage may seem to cure a backache entirely, since pain from the original source, such as a protruding disc, may have subsided in the meantime. You should keep in mind, however, that massage won't cure the trouble that brought on the spasm in the first place. And, of course, if that original condition causes more pain, you may be in for another spasm as well.

Manipulation, too, can be useful in loosening up muscles and joints tightened by a spasm. In fact, that is about all that manipulation is good for, as I pointed out in Chapter Seven. Manipulation doesn't always work, however, and it may hurt, especially if you have a pinched nerve. But hurt, remember, is not the same as harm; ordinarily you can't harm yourself this way. You'll be better off, just the same, if you apply the rule I mentioned earlier: no pain control remedy should make you feel worse. It may cause a new discomfort (remember, that's how liniment works), but it definitely should not increase the very pain you are trying to escape.

Craniosacral Therapy, Therapeutic Touch, and the Like

Whereas conventional spinal manipulation or adjustment may have a place in the management of acute mechanical low back pain, there is no validity to the claims of a number of practitioners who work beyond the fringe of medical science.

Craniosacral therapy purports to solve back problems by adjusting the relative positions of the bones in the skull. The fact that, in the adult, these bones are incapable of separate movement doesn't seem to interfere with the theory. The "sacral" part of the name arises from the belief that the body possesses a natural rhythm; six to twelve times a minute as your head grows larger, your spine grows shorter. As your head shrinks, your spine lengthens again. Changing this pattern is part of the therapy. Sound ridiculous? It's a multimillion-dollar business used to treat everything from projectile vomiting to learning disabilities.

Therapeutic touch is a bit of a misnomer. As a patient, you are not touched at all. The practitioner runs his or her hands over the contours of your body, sensing the electrical aura that is supposed to emanate from us all. Detecting a lack of flow within the aura, the therapist rapidly moves the hands in a manner designed to correct the problem. Using the same theory, I've tried waving my hands over the radio to improve the reception, but it has never worked for me.

Ultrasound

This is a modified version of the microwave oven. It can do one thing you can't do with your hot water bottle, poultices, or liniments: it can beam heat right into your body, well below the surface of your skin. And that may ease the pain in your spine. Or it may not. The whole idea, you see, is based on two assumptions — both of them unproven. One assumption is that the heat generated by ultrasound will actually reach the affected areas. No one can say for sure that it will. The second assumption is that heat eases pain. We know that heat causes blood vessels to expand and extra blood to accumulate. But does extra blood ease pain? Nobody knows. All we know, really, is that sometimes ultrasound helps a bad back feel better — at least for a while.

Magnetic Field Therapy

Another form of radiant energy used for back pain is magnetic. The device is a large ring that fits over the torso, or other affected area, and emits electromagnetic waves. Although the theory is obscure, these waves are considered to have healing properties, and the manufacturers claim relief for aching backs, aching feet, or just about any aching part. It's all a bit too slick for me. If magnetic waves can heal, then we should be getting much more than impressive pictures from magnetic resonance imaging; we should be curing a lot of disease. But we're not.

The TENS Machine and Interferential Currents

If the TENS machine didn't already exist, it might have to be invented to satisfy the backache victims who need to spend money on a magic box. TENS stands for Transcutaneous Electric Nerve Stimulation. The device is about the size of a small cassette player, costs considerably more, and comes with an impressive collection of wires and sticking pads. All you do is apply the pads over various sore spots and run the wires to the control unit in your shirt pocket or hanging from your belt. Then, no matter where you are when your back pain strikes, you can push a button or two and zap yourself with electrical impulses.

A variation on the same theme is the use of an interferential machine. It produces electrical currents administered to the skin through large pads that look vaguely like suction cups. Two electrical frequencies set up an interference pattern, hence the name, which acts in much the same way TENS does. Many patients say interferential is more comfortable, and it has the extra prestige of requiring professional application.

These devices are not fraudulent, although the reason for their effect is far from clear. There is reason to suppose that they trigger the release of pain-killing endorphins. Out of every ten people who try TENS for the first time, about seven enjoy beneficial results. The trouble is, it's easy to become emotionally dependent on that little black box. Meanwhile, your body becomes resistant to the impulses. And so, the more treatment you take, the more you need. Soon you need more than the machine can deliver. And of course TENS, even at its best, is just a pain-killer, not a cure. It won't do a thing to your bulging disc or your worn facet.

Worst of all, it encourages the Free Lunch Syndrome — the notion that you can heal your back easily, without expending any time or effort. You delegate your responsibility to the box and it does the job in an instant. Meanwhile, you shun the treatment you really need — the program of long-term care that demands a conscious effort, a degree of discomfort, and a measure of self-discipline.

Cold Laser Therapy

One particularly high-tech alternative to relieve back pain is cold laser therapy. It employs a complex and expensive machine to shine a laser on the affected area of the back. Laser (Light Amplification by Stimulated Emission of Radiation) produces a beam of light that travels in a perfectly straight line and can contain tremendous energy. A laser can signal satellites or burn holes in bricks, and it is used as a cutting tool in some surgery. But the cold laser has an extremely low energy concentration; it's the laser pointer I use in many of my lectures. Shone on the skin of the back, the laser effect is lost within millimeters of the surface, long before it could have any effect on the spine beneath. Because of this fact, I've heard advocates of laser therapy suggest it is the pure color of the light, rather than the energy content or the ability to travel in straight lines, that is important. They recommend one color laser for one problem and another color for something else. When I remembered that Newton showed that sunlight through a prism possessed all the colors of the

POULTICES, PULLEYS, AND PILLS   159

rainbow, I started asking patients if they wouldn't rather sit outside on a warm sunny day. It's a lot cheaper than laser and it should work just as well.

Muscle Relaxants

I often tell patients in the education classes at the Back Institute that there are no such things as muscle relaxants — only people relaxants. No matter what they're called, they can't be directed at a specific group of muscles. Taken orally, they have to relax the whole person.

If your doctor prescribes one of these drugs for you, it may not suit your lifestyle to be completely relaxed. It's hard to keep going when your brain feels as though it's covered with fuzz, and there can be a bit of a hangover the next morning. Muscle relaxants aren't pain relievers — not directly, anyway. About all that a relaxant can do for your back is loosen up a muscle spasm — assuming you have one — and thus indirectly reduce your pain.

Anti-inflammatory Drugs

Inflammation could be described as a speeded-up version of what is happening in your body all the time, with cells coming and going, being born and dying. The accelerated pace is one of your body's many defenses against injury, a quick means of removing unwanted substances and initiating repair. This process can slip out of control, and become painful. Anti-inflammatories are drugs that slow an abnormally rapid process to a normal pace. Aspirin in high dosages is probably the best known and most widely used anti-inflammatory of them all. The anti-inflammatories commonly prescribed by doctors fall into two classes: steroids and non-steroidal anti-inflammatory drugs.

Steroids, such as cortisone, may be taken by mouth for general effect or injected into discs, joints, or even the spinal canal to reduce unwanted local inflammation. There is no doubt that cortisone is capable of reducing inflammation, but the desired pain relief does not always occur. One reason may be that the pain is caused not by inflammation but by a mechanical condition that remains unchanged. Even when inflammation is apparently the cause of the pain, the cortisone may not work. Whenever a disc presses against a nerve, a complex chemical reaction takes place. The cortisone may take care of the inflammation but leave the physical pressure unaffected.

Even in instances where cortisone does reduce pain, it is only a stopgap measure, since it does nothing to remedy the cause of the pain. But stopgaps can be worthwhile if they are recognized and employed for what they are.

Non-steroidal anti-inflammatory drugs (NSAIDS) tend to offer an all-or-nothing proposition. When they work, they work well; in other cases, they seem to have no effect. Their success varies widely from patient to patient and even from one use to another for the same patient.

There are many non-steroidal drugs to choose from, and some enjoy a period of popularity and then fall out of favor. In spite of years of research, no one is sure just how the NSAIDS work. We know they have many methods of action, which would explain the wide variation in patient response, and we know that almost all have a negative effect on the stomach. One theory suggests that the normal function of the stomach is similar to continuous inflammation and by slowing down that reaction, NSAIDS upset the balance.

Non-steroidal anti-inflammatory drugs have a place. But they are powerful agents with a continuing risk of complications and they can do nothing to cure the mechanical problems caused by aging.

Stiffening Injections

Sad to say, it sometimes seems that if you look hard enough, you can find some doctor who will inject you with almost anything — just short of what's lethal — in the guise of treatment for your back. Such injections include sugar, salt water (dignified as "hypertonic saline"), and phenol (alias carbolic acid). There is no good scientific evidence to prove that any of these substances will help your back, either by relieving pain or by promoting healing — except, of course, by creating the Placebo Effect, which I discussed in Chapter Seven.

The proponents of such injections, however, are not easily troubled by their lack of scientific backing. They have their own theories. Injecting sugar into the spinal area, for example, is said to "tighten the ligaments" by causing inflammation that "scars down the joint and tightens it up." But nobody has ever established that back problems are caused by "loose joints" and that a back will get better if those joints are "tightened." Anyway, most inflammation doesn't cause tightening. Rather, it creates damage that allows ligaments to stretch and makes joints loose. It makes no sense that a reaction that works one way in the rest of the body should produce a completely different response in the back.

Another type of routine injection is the use of local anesthetic into sore spots — trigger points, they're called. The idea is simply to stop pain by freezing the painful location, the way your dentist might freeze a painful tooth. Of course, the dentist would then go on to fill the cavity or pull the tooth. Practitioners of pain-relieving injections often do nothing at all, except invite you back for another needle when the anesthetic wears off. It's a treatment that focuses on pain and, as we have already seen, sustaining a pain focus for someone with chronic back problems is poor therapy.

And these injections can cost hundreds of dollars — paid by patients who reason that if something is expensive, it must be good. A few doctors willing to nurture that notion are making a full-time specialty out of questionable practices.

Rhizotomy

Also known as rhizolysis, this treatment remains popular with very few doctors. The term means to cut or destroy a nerve root. This operation involves cutting the nerves to the facet joints. It sounds perfectly logical: since the facet is a common site of back pain, depriving the joint of its ability to feel pain should cure your trouble. But the theory doesn't work out in practice. Your body is not deterred that easily from doing its normal job of transmitting sensations. When one route is cut off, another is used. The operation may be a complete success — except that the patient's back still hurts. In some cases, the surgeon fails to cut all the nerves involved. In an attempt to make it more effective, the original surgical approach has been replaced largely by nerve destruction employing either a radio-frequency probe or thermal or chemical means. Still, the success for rhizotomy, even with the newest techniques, remains about thirty percent, less than the anticipated Placebo Effect.

Chemonucleolysis

Translated from Doctor, chemonucleolysis means a chemical destruction of the disc center. This is a controversial form of back treatment. The procedure, intended to relieve the pressure exerted on a nerve by a bulging disc, consists of injecting the disc with an enzyme related to the enzyme used in those meat tenderizers you sprinkle on tough steaks. Injected into a bulging disc, it apparently denatures the protein, thereby drying out the nuclear material.

Chemonucleolysis can be a painful treatment, even when administered under heavy sedation, but it takes less time, is less painful, has fewer complications, and causes less aggravation than surgery, which should be the alternative.

Unfortunately, chemonucleolysis is unpredictable, sometimes providing relief within minutes, at other times not for weeks, and sometimes not at all. The overall success in treating acute disc herniations with nerve-root involvement is about seventy percent.

Chemonucleolysis can have side effects. The most serious is an allergic reaction that can be fatal. This reaction, however, is immediately evident, making the risk very slight for any patient under competent medical supervision.

My opinion of chemical disc destruction is that it's safe enough but is useful only in treating a patient who has a herniated disc pressing on a nerve. It is of no use in patients with disc pain (Pattern One), facet pain (Pattern Two), or bony pressure (Pattern Four). And that is my biggest objection. The procedure is useful only for patients with acutely pinched nerves — fewer than one in every ten people with common backache. Since most of this small group gets better with less aggressive treatment, probably one person in a hundred requires the enzyme injection. The same ratio is true for surgery, but because the needle is far simpler than the knife, it gets used far more readily. And far too often, in my view.

At the beginning of this chapter, I remarked on the wide range of choices open to any patient in search of a remedy for back pain. Like any back doctor, I hope that, as we learn more about the physiology and pathology of back problems, many of the inconsistent and limited treatments will be made reliable and more effective, and that, with better understanding, the worthless "cures" will disappear.

At the moment, however, reliable, medically proven remedies beyond those used for short-term pain relief, are limited to a group of standard surgical procedures, plus the conservative treatment — the exercise, the good postural habits, and the improved lifestyle — on which the philosophy of this book is based.

As you will learn in the next chapter, surgery is not "the ultimate" in back treatment but merely a means of helping to correct certain conditions that arise in the spines of a minority of back patients. And, as you will see from later chapters, surgery is no substitute for a lifelong program of sensible back care.

10 Surgery: When, Why, and How?

To many people with back problems, spinal surgery is magic — the cure-all for any condition too serious to be remedied by some "lesser" treatment.

That belief, however, has no basis in reality. For one thing, it ignores the fact that surgery is capable of helping only a fraction of all backache victims. And, among the relatively few who can benefit from surgery, it encourages unrealistic expectations of a complete, life-long cure.

The concept of surgery as a cure-all is sometimes nurtured by doctors themselves. In a well-meaning attempt to encourage a positive attitude toward an impending operation, a surgeon may speak too glibly of "getting you all fixed up" or "taking care of your disc trouble."

It sounds straightforward, but no back operation can be unconditionally guaranteed. And even if it could, your back problems would not necessarily be over for all time. Some disc or joint that never caused trouble before could start hurting next week or next year. In any case, spinal surgery can't really cure a bad back — at least not in the sense that an appendectomy can cure appendicitis. Spinal surgery can correct a specific mechanical condition, such as a bulging disc pressing against a nerve. But in doing so, it will leave you with a back that is something less than normal. A normal back, as I have said before, doesn't have a scar on it. And, whatever condition is being corrected, you are almost certain to come out with some part of your spine removed or some once-movable joint permanently immobilized. In fact, as we'll see later in this chapter, the alterations that surgery creates in your spine may even cause or contribute to new back trouble. I'm not opposed to spinal surgery. On the contrary, as an orthopedic surgeon with a particular interest in spine, I perform back operations every week. What I am saying is that surgery has limitations that many back patients fail to appreciate.

Patients also fail, sometimes, to understand why a doctor will recommend surgery in a given case. They'll tell their friends, "My back was so painful he just had to operate." Actually, the degree of pain is only one factor in the decision to operate. There is also a widely held notion that surgery is a means of "getting it all over with quickly" and avoiding the need for further back care. The fact is that when you are left with a less-than-normal back, you will have more reason than ever to keep it in condition with exercise and proper living habits. I expect your ability to return to normal, yet your back will never be exactly the same.

In deciding whether to operate, your doctor must answer one basic question: "Does this patient have a condition that can be — and should be — corrected by surgery?" In other words, surgery is not a substitute for other forms of treatment; like any other, it should be used when it is the most appropriate treatment in the circumstances, and it should be rejected when it is not. Surgery is always specific; it is never a last resort.

Whenever that point seems to escape one of my patients, I draw the analogy of the sick tree. If something is ailing a favorite tree in your front yard, you wouldn't expect to make it well automatically by lopping off a branch or two. You'd try to find out was wrong and apply the appropriate remedy, whether it was a splint to heal a serious break, or a wire fence to protect the bark from hungry porcupines. You'd use surgery only when surgery was the best or only solution. Often I extend the analogy to emphasize the need for long-term care. I point out that the immediate remedy for that tree would be no substitute for its continuing needs — water, fertilizer, sunlight, and space in which to grow.

As long as you realize that surgery is just one step in the lifelong management of your back, you are unlikely to be disappointed by the outcome of an operation. In many cases, surgery produces some exciting results, such as the instant relief of pain, following the removal of a large chunk of disc resting against a nerve root. But it is a mistake to think of spinal surgery as a measure that will inevitably end in either triumph or tragedy. Usually the outcome will lie somewhere between these two extremes.

Having acquired realistic expectations, you can increase your chance of success even more by learning everything you can about the physical aspects of your operation: why surgery is a good idea in your case, how you can prepare yourself for it, what your doctor will do in the operating room, how you'll feel afterward, and what you can do to help ensure a speedy recovery. Chances are, you will have plenty of time to learn everything you need to know. For, with the exception of an acute cauda equina syndrome (which I described in Chapter Eight), a decision to operate on your spine won't be made overnight. Or let me put it another way: if your doctor makes a snap decision about surgery for you, I suggest you make a snap decision and request a second opinion from another surgeon.

A number of years ago, a forty-three-year-old warehouseman came to me from another doctor who had recommended surgery. My patient had wrenched his back while lifting a heavy food carton in a supermarket warehouse. By the time I saw him, he had been back on the job for two months. But occasionally, his spine still hurt, especially at the end of a day's work.

His first doctor — call him Dr. M. — had x-rayed his back and produced a diagnosis that I believe was accurate: the man had spondylolysis. That's the condition where small fractures remain in the ridges of bones separating the facet joints on the back of a vertebra. The result is an abnormal separation between the upper and lower sets of joints on the back of that one bone.

Research has shown that this condition usually appears before the age of five. My patient, then, had had these defects in his spine for more than thirty-five years. Yet he had never had back pain until the day of that minor accident in the warehouse.

I'm sure Dr. M. would agree with me that those were the facts of the case. But on the question of surgery we parted company. Dr. M. believed that fusion was an urgent necessity, to bring stability to those separated joints.

That isn't the way I saw it. Here was a man whose spondylolysis had given him no trouble whatever for thirty-five years or more. Now his first attack of pain was subsiding and could probably be remedied entirely if someone showed him the basics of back care and proper lifting techniques. In my opinion, surgery was hardly necessary, let alone urgent.

What's more, the patient himself didn't want the operation. He was more than willing to try a program of exercise and activity adjustment. And so that's what I prescribed for him. I saw my patient recently, at a hockey game. He is still doing his exercises and his back is fine. He has everything to gain and nothing to lose. If the care program is effective, he will never need surgery. On the other hand, if surgery proves to be necessary after all, he will be well prepared for it — thoroughly briefed and trained in the self-help measures that are vital in the postoperative period.

His situation brings to mind another misconception people often have about back treatment. Patients assume that when a surgeon, me for example, declines to operate, there is nothing more I can do for them. Actually, I can provide several other major services. I can examine your back and diagnose your problem. I can direct the conservative management. I can prescribe medication for you. I can initiate and review your rehabilitation program. And I can monitor your condition, conducting additional examinations and altering the treatment whenever it seems wise to do so.

The limitations of surgery become clear once you learn that there are only two basic kinds of operations for coping with common back trouble. One involves decompression; the other stabilization.

In plainer English, decompression means relieving the pressure that part of the spine is exerting on the spinal nerves. There are two types of patients who require decompressive surgery — those with a disc pressing on a nerve, and those with a nerve being squeezed by the bone itself. Most often a bulging disc is responsible for pressure on a nerve, typically against a nerve root where it leaves the spine. The pressure may occur within the canal or, as we saw earlier, a piece of the disc may break away and lodge against a nerve in the exit tunnel. These are both causes of Pattern Three back trouble. In other cases, with Pattern Four, where decompression is required, the culprit is not a disc but a bony prominence that is squeezing down on a nerve or closing the canal. Surgery here removes the offending portion of bone and opens the space around the nerve to allow resumption of normal circulation.

Surgery to relieve disc pressure entails removal of part of the disc. This operation is known conventionally, but not accurately, as a disc removal or, in Doctor, a discotomy. Removal of bone covering the nerve is termed a laminectomy. Since "-otomy" means to cut a hole, discotomy means to cut a hole in a disc. And since "-ectomy" means "the removal of," "laminectomy" means the removal of the lamina, the roof of the spinal canal. Most of the back operations I perform are either discotomies or laminectomies. (Incidentally, if part of the bone on the back of the spinal canal is cut away just to allow room for the removal of a bulging disc, the operation gains the impressive title of hemilaminectomy-discotomy.) Microdiscotomy is a term describing the removal of a portion of a disc with the aid of an operating microscope. There is nothing wrong with this technique, but I believe a good surgeon can do his job just as well with a conventional pair of magnifying glasses.

Stabilization means eliminating movement at one or more spinal level. This is done by a process called fusion — that is, joining bones on each side of the disc. Typically, fusion is performed at the level of a disc whose shock-absorbing function has failed or of a badly worn and painful joint that fails to improve with time and exercise. Occasionally, more than one level may be fused, but the risk of failure increases with each additional level.

Whenever he decides to operate for common back trouble, a surgeon will always have decompression, stabilization, or both as his objective. Although you may hear someone with back trouble talking about having an exploratory operation, it is not quite as it sounds. Before he operates, a surgeon can usually learn all he needs to know about your back problem from your history, your physical examination, and whatever x-rays and tests are appropriate. No competent surgeon will open your back just to poke around in search of trouble, although he may need to explore one small area to actually see the problem. No incision can provide a view of more than a fraction of your total spine. By the time he takes scalpel in hand, your surgeon has to know exactly where he's going and what he expects to do when he gets there.

By now, you may be wondering what convinces a doctor that one particular back patient needs a surgical decompression when so many others don't. One important clue is the patient's failure to respond to conservative management — rest, exercise, and proper habits. I would judge this not only from the continuing pain the patient describes but also from the persistence of weaknesses in the muscles, loss of reflexes, and decreased sensation in parts of the legs.

Surgery is also called for when a patient has a loss of motor power that could be described as either massive or progressive. I call a defect massive if, for example, the person has lost all power to stand on tiptoe because she is unable to move her foot downward. And certainly I would call a defect progressive if a minor weakness developed into a major one in only a few weeks' time, despite proper conservative care. It's rare to see either a massive or a progressive loss of nerve function, but when either appears, I recommend early surgery.

Sometimes I conclude that surgery is necessary when I see a patient who responds to conservative management for a few months but who continues to suffer repeated attacks of back and leg pain with loss of function in the same muscles or nerves each time. The decision to operate in this case is a judgment call on my part. It is based on my assessment of the disruption of the patient's life by the recurrent attacks and by my opinion of the patient's ability to cope with each episode of back pain. That's unscientific, I know, but much of healing is still an art, not a science, and sometimes there is nothing better than sound clinical judgment based on experience.

Apart from specific diseases and serious back injuries (which this book is not intended to cover), the only other condition that would prompt me to undertake decompressive back surgery is a central disc herniation. This is the extremely rare condition I described in Chapter Eight: a protruding disc exerts pressure on several nerves inside the spinal canal. This is the only diagnosis in the realm of low back pain that may require an immediate operation.

Let us suppose that you are a patient of mine in need of a discotomy. Here's what you can expect.

You will have most of your tests as an outpatient. If you require a myelogram or a CT myelogram, it may be done after your admission to hospital for surgery, but more and more even these invasive procedures are performed on an outpatient basis. On the afternoon before your surgery, you come into hospital to be examined and have your history taken by one of the hospital doctors, who will order routine blood and urine tests if they have not been done already. You may receive preoperative instruction from the nursing staff. The night before your operation, you will be given a sedative and instructed to not eat or drink anything after midnight. Some hospitals, mine included, may even allow you to remain at home until the morning of your operation. All the tests and education before surgery will be done prior to admission. It's a cost saving, but more importantly, many people handle their anxiety about the operation better at home.

On the morning of your surgery, you will be given a needle to relax you before you are transferred to the operating room. There, you are put under a general anesthetic and positioned face down over a special frame on the operating table. Now you can breathe easily and your back is readily accessible.

I begin your discotomy by making a 1-inch (2.5 cm) incision over your spine in your low back. If necessary, I use x-ray to check the exact location of my cut. Then I work my way slowly downward by moving through or around the various layers of muscle, bone, and ligament I encounter along the way. After removing one small part of the roof of the spinal canal, I arrive at the nerve root and finally the disc.

If there are any loose fragments of the disc evident, I remove them. I look for the weak spot or hole I know will be found in the shell of the disc, much like a blowout in a tire, from which some of the contents may have escaped. The outer part of the disc is highly elastic. Once a fragment of the nucleus has pushed through, the tear may close. In that case, I leave the shell alone and let your body get started with healing. If the rent is large enough, I will probe the inside of the disc, which is often surprisingly empty, to be sure there are no other loose pieces. I will leave the disc empty, confident that over the next several weeks the space will become partly and painlessly occupied by scar tissue.

Withdrawal is much easier than the entry was: I simply replace the nerve root and muscles that have been temporarily pushed aside, bring the incision together, and stitch up the skin.

The whole operation, from opening to closing, takes less than an hour.

You are taken to the recovery room where you regain consciousness. When most of the effects of the anesthetic

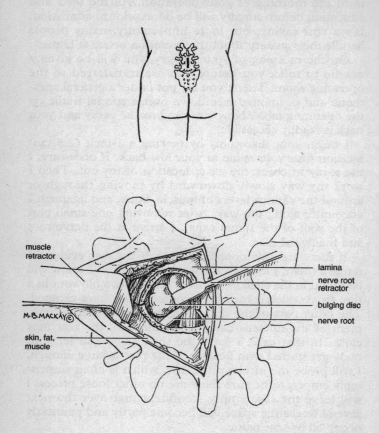

muscle
retractor

lamina

nerve root
retractor

bulging disc

nerve root

M.B.MACKAY©

skin, fat,
muscle

Fig. 16. This illustration represents the surgeon's view of the
back during a disc operation at the L4-5 level. With a small
part of the roof removed, little is visible within the spinal
canal except a single nerve root and the bulging portion of the
disc.

have worn off, you are returned to your own room in the hospital. Once you are fully awake, I expect you to get out of bed and start walking. The sooner the better. You can go home as soon as you want, often within the first twenty-four hours. For a couple of days, your back will be sore. The discomfort will come mainly from your back muscles, which were unavoidably bruised when I pushed them aside. But soon you realize that this new pain represents a good trade-off. It's not nearly so sharp or troublesome as the pain from a pinched nerve. That horrible pain down your leg is gone. And, best of all, the pain you have now is temporary.

You may find, though, that your stomach has stopped working. This is probably due to your position on the operating table and the effect of the anesthetic. I will have you avoid solid food until your digestive tract is functioning normally again.

Most people are surprised to find that no special precautions are necessary to keep their backs from "falling apart." Standing, leaning, or lying down are much easier on the soft tissues than sitting, but you have my permission to do anything you want; I always exclude sky-diving and show jumping. The pressure on the nerve is gone and in most cases it won't be back. You may feel a few twinges or shocks as the nerve gets used to its new freedom, but they rapidly disappear.

At home, you will feel you need extra rest. Although the operating time is short and the recovery is rapid, back surgery is a great strain on your system. Rest is good, but activity is better, and a frequent mix of both is best of all.

No special appliances, equipment, or therapy are necessary during your convalescence. Your own bed is fine. You won't wear a brace. I recommend patients return to regular supervised exercise within a week of surgery. There is nothing you need to fear, and the guidance and reassurance of the physiotherapist will help build your confidence. Depending on what you do for a living, I will suggest you go back to work in four to six weeks after the operation. Many patients return much sooner. One patient, who supervised the construction of new clinics for CBI, was at his desk the morning after surgery. A well-known entertainer returned to his concert tour of North America four days after his back operation and celebrated the six-week anniversary by sinking his first hole in one.

The discotomy is the least disruptive kind of major back surgery, and it has a ninety percent chance of being a complete success — no more pain or trouble from that disc.

I said earlier that decompression operations don't necessarily involve discs. Especially in older patients, the bone of the vertebra can exert pressure on a nerve root. It may be an unusually narrow spinal canal or the partial closing of the nerve's exit between two adjacent vertebrae. In some cases, a bone spur on the edge of a facet joint may press the nerve against the floor of the exit tunnel.

Another variation occurs after a disc has narrowed and allowed the vertebrae to settle together more closely than normal. This creates an abnormally sharp angle in the nerve at its point of exit. The result is the same sort of pinching effect that occurs when you try to haul a garden hose around the corner of your house.

Nerve pressure may develop in people whose spinal canal has grown too narrow from the natural bony overgrowth of aging or has never developed to normal size in the first place. In either case, the nerves of the canal have no room, and the cramped quarters reduce their supply of blood, making it impossible for the patient to walk more than a short distance without stopping to rest, the typical picture of Pattern Four pain.

With all these various conditions, the general surgical approach is a decompression operation of the same type as for a herniated disc. The surgeon removes a section of bone or enlarges an exit canal, depending on what is exerting pressure on the nerve, but he usually leaves the disc intact. In a case of spinal canal narrowing, all the roof and inner portions of the joint are usually removed. The decompression is very effective when only one level is involved. Enlarging the canal in more than three verte-brae often gives disappointing results.

If you were to have one of these bony decompression operations, your routine during recovery and convales-cence would likely be the same as after a standard disco-tomy, although the pace is generally slower. Because more of the spine must be exposed, more muscle is pushed aside and bruised, and there is more postopera-tive back pain.

Fusions of two or more vertebrae are performed less frequently than simple decompressions. As a rule, a number of factors must come together before I will rec-ommend fusion for any patient. Fusion, you see, is usual-ly a judgment call. Before I perform this operation on anyone, I have to be convinced that the person has Pattern One or Pattern Two back pain that cannot be controlled by non-operative measures, and that the mag-nitude of the problem has rendered the patient incapable of work or even routine daily activities.

The patient's attitude and past record must also be right. I must be convinced that she has made a serious, prolonged attempt to remedy her condition through a program of exercise and good living habits. I consider six months of strenuous back fitness exercise to be a mini-mum requirement for consideration of surgery. The patient must realize that fusion won't make the spine normal. She must acknowledge the importance of post-operative care — indefinitely. She must be prepared to accept a degree of postoperative discomfort, if not pain. If anyone comes to me with a mild backache and wants a fusion so there will be no backache at all, I can't help. And, finally, she must have confidence in me as her sur-geon. She must believe that what I do will make her feel better, even though I can't offer to cure her.

If we're lucky, the problem will prove to be confined to a single level. That way, our chances of success are greatest. If only a single level has to be fused, we have over a ninety percent chance of fusing it successfully. If two levels are fused at the same operation, the percentage drops to roughly eighty. With three levels, we are down to a success rate near seventy percent. It's a matter of simple mechanics: the greater the length of the spine involved, the less chance we have of immobilizing it entirely against the stress of normal movement.

If age and wear have damaged more than three levels, the problem is generally beyond surgical correction. In other circumstances, such as cases of spinal curvature (scoliosis), surgeons sometimes fuse as many as eight or ten levels. Such operations, however, are performed for very different reasons and usually in a much younger age group. The effects of years of hard use on all the discs and joints in the low back cannot be neutralized or reversed by any operative procedure.

Let's suppose now that you are a patient who is to undergo a spinal fusion. Here's what happens. You go through the same preliminaries as you would for a discotomy, and I begin with essentially the same kind of incision, except that it is longer. I clear away more muscle and other material than I would to treat a disc, and I thoroughly clean off the backs and bony projections of the vertebrae that are to be fused.

Now I roughen the exposed surfaces of these vertebrae with a power burr. This deliberate damage activates the bone's healing response and leads to fusion.

Through either the same incision or a separate one, I expose the back of your pelvis, which will provide me with the extra bone I need. I carve off little strips of bone a bit thicker than matchsticks, each about an inch (2.5 cm) long, or I employ a hollow power reamer to grind up and collect the bone in a form that resembles wet beach sand. I pack the bone meal or the matchsticks on each side of the vertebrae, bridging the gap from one bone to the next.

In roughening the back surfaces of the vertebrae, I stimulate the body into reacting as though a fracture had occurred. The body's healing mechanism incorporates the newly placed bone sticks or paste into the spine, as though they are parts of vertebrae that have broken away.

If the fusion works as well as it should, the bone I add will soon be united to the separate vertebrae, joining them into a solid section.

In many cases, I add some type of metal fixation to immobilize the bones. Screws are inserted within the walls of the nerve tunnel and advanced into the drum-shaped vertebral body. The screws are linked together with a rod or plate to form a rigid frame. Many patients and a few surgeons are fascinated by the idea of putting metallic implants into the spine. This emphasis on hardware obscures a fundamental fact: fusion comes from the bone, not from the plates and screws. They are only the clamps that hold two pieces of wood together while the glue sets. If the glue doesn't stick, the project is a failure. If the vertebrae don't unite, the metal will always fail.

As I withdraw from the site, I replace any muscles that have been pushed aside, then close the skin incision in a routine manner. If I have made a separate incision at the pelvis, of course I close it too.

During the postoperative period, you will treat your spine more carefully than you would have done after a simple discotomy. The incision is much longer and the muscles are a lot more painful. Although I don't use one, some surgeons will require you to wear a brace for several weeks after the surgery to restrict your movement. The idea is to give the new bone a chance to heal without disruption, to attach firmly to the adjacent vertebrae. Bony consolidation is visible on x-ray in about six weeks, but will not be complete for up to two years.

You will be able to leave hospital a few days after surgery. I suggest you begin gentle exercises like walking as soon as you can and start a formal physical training routine about two months after the operation.

Oddly, the sorest part of your body is often not the site of the fusion but the donor site — an area in your pelvic bone where the bone for the bone graft was obtained. Pain in this area can persist for six months or more.

Occasionally I perform a spinal fusion in the low back by operating from the front of the patient's body. This may be necessary if a solid fusion cannot be achieved from behind; for example, when previous surgery has removed most of the bone covering the spinal cord and there is no way of positioning the bone graft. The approach from the front allows me to remove much of the disc and to pack the space between the vertebrae with bone sticks I have obtained from the pelvis. Some type of metallic internal fixation is usually required. Packing bone between the vertebral bodies can also be accomplished from behind by retracting the nerves and working through the spinal canal.

Surgery from the front of the spine is standard for operations on discs in the cervical or neck area. This approach is used for the neck because, unlike the low back, where nerves in the spinal canal can be pushed aside to allow access to the disc space, the cervical spine contains a section of the spinal cord that cannot be moved. Discotomy in the neck is routinely combined with fusion because this part of the spine might otherwise become unstable.

Many patients assume that a fusion will make their backs stronger than normal. In fact, fusion simply makes your back more rigid — and not even as effectively as nature does more gradually and more subtly. Fusion is an awkward arrangement that inevitably increases the strain on the unfused levels nearby. This extra load can lead to problems in the future. And, as we saw, the greater the number of vertebrae we attempt to fuse, the greater the chance of failure through mechanical stress. You may be asked to consider having a fusion for common back pain from wear in a disc or joint. The more levels your surgeon wants to fuse, the more skeptical you should be, and the more inclined to seek a second opinion.

Because of the complications associated with conventional spine surgery, a number of new procedures have attracted interest. Decompressions are being done by means of a small tube passed through the skin into the disc. The center of the disc is removed with a mechanical cutting device or vaporized with a laser (this is not cold laser therapy). These techniques do not specifically attack the disc fragment pressing on the nerve. The idea is that with a large hole in the middle of the disc, the offending piece will fall back inside. Unfortunately, there is no proof this happens, and the results of these treatments are extremely inconsistent. Some surgeons are approaching the problem directly by operating through a scope much like the one used for arthroscopic knee surgery.

The problems after fusion have spurred a great deal of research on the artificial disc. Metal, plastic, and a number of new jelly-like substances have been tried. None has yet proven uniformly successful.

Whether you have had a stabilization or a decompression, the time may come when your doctor recommends a second operation on your spine. If that happens, you have every right to know why. The key question is: Is this a new problem, or are we just trying to correct trouble left over from the first time? Here are some explanations you may hear and my comments.

"The same disc is causing trouble again."

This doesn't happen often. The recurrence rate after surgery is less than five percent. And it will be a new, unrelated event following a minimum of six, and preferably twelve, months of pain relief from the first surgery. The treatment for a new herniation at the old surgical site is no different than if there had been no previous operation. That means surgery doesn't come first. Start again with simple pain control techniques and stretching exercise.

"A different disc has herniated."

That's just bad luck. If conservative management doesn't yield results, surgery may be the only solution. This is also true if the same disc has now herniated on the opposite side and is affecting the opposite leg. But a successful first operation is not a justification for rushing into a second one.

"Your problem is that there's scarring on the nerve root."

Scar tissue is the natural result of surgery. Some scar is inevitable, and some people scar more aggressively than others. Since surgery produces scar tissue, using an operation to remove it is a poor choice. When scar is removed, more will form.

"That same nerve is being pinched again. Last time the disc was to blame; this time it's the bone."

This is plausible. When a disc loses some of its contents and height, the vertebrae come together more closely and the nerve exit is narrowed. A portion of the bone may be pressing down on the nerve. Your doctor may recommend either a bony decompression to relieve the pressure or a fusion to prevent further narrowing of the joint. Or both. But don't blame your first operation for your new trouble; it might have occurred anyway.

"The fusion didn't hold."

To be more precise, the fusion didn't take; the glue didn't stick. There is almost a ten percent chance that even a one-level fusion will fail. But before you consent to a second attempt at fusing the same level, make sure you receive clear and positive answers to these three questions: 1. Has my fusion really failed, or is it only my continuing back pain that is demanding surgery? 2. Is that failed fusion clearly the site of my pain? 3. Is my pain actually caused by movement at that level, so that a successful fusion will produce relief?

"The fusion is solid — your pain must be coming from somewhere else."

That's not necessarily true. A solid fusion does not guarantee freedom from back pain. New levels can be affected, but pain may come from scar tissue or nerve entrapment in the fused area, and it is difficult to tell from x-rays whether a fusion is really solid.

Incidentally, I have seen the opposite situation — where the fusion failed but the patient's back pain was relieved. How does this happen? Nobody knows.

"Your present fusion is fine, but now the level next to it is wearing out."

Unfortunately, this one is all too likely. It points up the fact that one fusion may lead to another. With one level immobilized, the adjacent discs and joints feel extra strain. This can be a problem, but it's one that cannot be avoided if the original fusion was necessary.

If you've had one successful fusion already, the question of having a second one requires serious thought. Consider carefully the amount of pain you're having, whether you've given conservative management a fair try, and whether the benefits are likely to be worth a second round of surgery, recovery, and convalescence.

Here's a good rule to remember when considering surgery: Your first chance is your best chance, your second chance is your last chance.

I hope these comments on second operations will prove enlightening to many readers besides those who have already had surgery or who are now considering it. If nothing else, the points I have raised now must surely emphasize that, far from being a magic cure-all, surgery can, in fact, become a source of new trouble and pain that might have been avoided.

At the same time, I don't want to overstate the case against surgery. In my opinion, the backlash in recent years against "too much surgery" — a popular criticism voiced frequently in magazines and newspapers — has been carried to an unjustified extreme. I believe it has hampered the healing of many afflictions, including back problems, because patients or their families have withheld their consent for the wrong reasons. After all, it is just as wrong to reject surgery that is needed as it is to propose surgery that is unnecessary.

If the need for spinal surgery is clear, proceed in the knowledge that, as long as you are in capable hands, the success rate in cases like yours is excellent. But if the picture is muddy, perhaps the wisest decision you can make is to discover for yourself whether your back problem will respond well to the program of conservative management set out in the next three chapters.

11 *Can You Spare Ten Minutes a Day?*

How would you like to know that you will never have another moment of serious worry about back pain?

That may sound like the sort of opening you would hear from some snake-oil salesman making a pitch for Professor Hamilton Hall's Miraculous Elixir for Bad Backs. But that's hardly what I'm selling. I am talking not about curing back pain but about controlling it and no longer fearing it. And certainly there are no miracles involved in my method. In fact, its most obvious weakness — if you can call it that — lies in its most undramatic simplicity. It is so simple that many people refuse, at first, to believe that it works.

But it does work. I know, because over the years I've seen the results in thousands of people who have attended the Canadian Back Institute and discovered how to manage their back problems, reducing their pain and overcoming their fears.

If they can achieve those results, so can you. You can begin, as they did, by recognizing that common backache is not a disease but a sign of normal wear that accompanies growth and maturity — like gray hair. Obviously, if you don't want the gray in your hair to show, you wouldn't go around looking for a cure for aging or for graying; you would accept the inevitability of it all and apply treatments to control your hair color. Similarly, if your back is suffering from the effects of age, you would be wise to learn about the condition, forget about finding a cure, and go to work on treatments that will enable you to control the pain.

183

You will soon discover that conservative management does not mean sparing your back at all costs and behaving like an invalid. It means taking charge of your spinal resources — building them up and then expanding them as you see fit, to suit your individual wants and needs. How do you lay the groundwork? By adopting what I call the Four A program of back pain management.

Attitude

Nothing is more important than understanding your back problem, knowing how to cope with an attack, and becoming confident that there is no longer anything to fear.

Accountability

You are responsible for the control of your own back pain. No one can do it for you and it's a mistake to let someone try. Sure you need help — that's what this book is all about — but the responsibility for solving the problem and getting on with a normal life belongs to you.

Activities of daily living

ADL, for short, need adjustment. They demand a change of lifestyle, but no sacrifice, on your part. You learn how to carry yourself and use your body in dozens of everyday situations — at work, play, recreation, and rest. Soon, the comfortable way becomes more natural for you than the pain-producing way.

Action

It takes about ten minutes a day to practice the pain control actions that can abolish your current pain and reduce your chances of having a disabling attack in the future. The type of simple exercise you require depends upon your particular pattern of pain, as we will see. The routines include stretching for rapid pain control and strengthening for lasting relief.

Since some back-sparing movements impose an added strain on leg muscles that may be unaccustomed to it, you might want to add a couple of thigh-strengthening exercises to your regular routine.

As I said, the program is simple. But it is not effortless. If you want to control your back problem instead of allowing it to control you, you must expend some effort. You must do the exercises faithfully throughout the day, and you must make good postural habits as routine as brushing your teeth or tying your shoelaces (both of which should be done with good posture). You will choose between flexion (forward-bending) exercises and extension (backward-bending) routines. Your decision is based on which movements normally reproduce your typical pain. With Pattern One, it hurts to bend forward, so you develop an extension program. If you have Pattern Two, your best chance for relief comes with flexion. Sounds too obvious, but there are no inside secrets. Whatever you do, keep it up and stick to a regular routine of about ten minutes a day. You must be patient, and you must persevere. You may gain short-term pain relief within days, or even hours, but lasting control takes much longer. Forget about medical miracles. Settle in for a long haul. Don't worry: there will be a pay-off, but it will take time — usually two or three months.

Adopting the right attitude does not mean brainwashing yourself. Rather, it means understanding the realities of back pain and knowing the appropriate responses. It's important, for example, to expect bad days as well as good ones, and to treat the bad days for what they are — just momentary setbacks, not the beginning of a steady decline.

And you must expect new attacks of back pain. But once you are prepared for them, you can look forward to reducing their severity and duration. If you used to have two attacks a year, you may well continue to have two attacks a year. But it's unlikely that your future attacks will be the "killers" that once prodded you with pain for a month or more. Instead, you may reduce them to mild episodes that are gone in a few days.

Although we speak of this program of self-treatment as conservative management, it is based on a philosophy of permissiveness. It may sound strange to hear someone talking about conservative treatment in one breath and permissiveness in the next, but the two fit together perfectly in this program. The idea is that you learn only principles and guidelines, not rules. It's up to you to decide what you want to do to conserve your spinal resources and how you want to expend them. The process is like putting money into a savings account and then budgeting the funds according to your needs, wants, or whims. Every time you exercise certain muscles or adopt a correct sitting posture, you're making a "deposit" in your "back account." Every time you subject your spine to unusual strain or fail to exercise it, you're making a "withdrawal."

Sometimes you may feel it's worthwhile to make a deliberate withdrawal — to endure a little pain in return for the advantage of carrying out a necessary task or a favorite activity. And why not? It won't harm you; at worst, it may just leave your back feeling sore for a day or two. You're probably better off playing in that golf tournament next Sunday and collecting a little back pain than you would be sitting at home missing the fun and feeling sorry for yourself. And go ahead and give a piggyback ride to that favorite niece you haven't seen for a year; she's worth a little discomfort, isn't she?

I take that attitude with me onto the basketball court. I've had Pattern One back pain since I was a teenager, but I love basketball. I know that every time I play the game my back will be stressed repeatedly, and I know perfectly well my back will be sore afterward. But so what? Hurt is not the same as harm. To me, it's a price worth paying for a good workout on the court — a fair trade-off that I make willingly. Perhaps you'll want to think a little more about trade-offs of your own, especially when you read Chapter 13 and see the effects various sports have on sore backs.

At the Canadian Back Institute, our treatment program is specialized. We divide it into three parts, called Stage I, Stage II, and Stage III. Stage I, the stage I discuss in most detail here, addresses pain control. Our therapists divide Stage I into three smaller parts: confirming that the chosen routine is correct; ensuring that the patient incorporates proper pain control exercises into his or her normal routine; and, finally, abolishing the pain. We have learned that there are three usual reasons for patients' failure to improve: they don't do the exercises, they do the exercises incorrectly, or they don't avoid temporarily the activities that bring on the pain. Of course, there is always the chance that the treatment direction is wrong and needs to be changed, but the first three reasons are far more common.

The pain control maneuvers you choose in Stage I depend on your pattern of pain. Before you start, review the patterns again. If you make a wrong choice, don't worry. You may increase your typical pain for a short while but you can't harm your back.

The exercises in Stage I are generally stretching routines. They can have an almost immediate effect, so use them frequently, a minute at a time, ten times a day. For most back pain sufferers, the first stage is measured in days. Once the pain can be controlled, you are ready to move on to Stage II.

The second stage focuses on recovery of movement that may have been lost during the acute attack. It's difficult to return to a normal life with a stiff back. In this stage, I encourage patients to begin moving in all directions, even the ones that cause typical pain. The idea is to recover a normal range, to make your back do everything it could do before. Use your pain control exercises whenever you need them, but the goal is a return to your normal back movement. Like Stage I, it may take only a few days.

Stage III lasts much longer. It is the stage of physical conditioning, regaining strength in the trunk and abdominal muscles, and improving muscle power in the legs. The pain control exercises should be second nature by now, and you can concentrate on a strengthening routine that gives you the best chance of reducing or even eliminating future attacks. Stage III can take months, but what have you got to lose? You look and feel better, and your back pain is finally under control.

Unlike a general fitness routine that conditions your various muscles and organs from head to toe, our plan is designed strictly to provide you with good control of your back. Fitness is important, and I recommend a general exercise program to anyone who is interested. Back exercise is not the same thing, and substitutions are not acceptable. If you want to work out two hours a day, fine, but be sure that a definite part of that time is set aside for your back program. That way, if fitness becomes a bore and the two hours are put to a different use, your back exercises stand a better chance of remaining a part of your daily routine.

Before you attempt a program of back exercise, make sure you understand its purpose. Exercise is one means of controlling your back pain and helping prevent future attacks. Exercise has a limited role for pain control in Pattern Three, the pinched nerve from a bulging disc. For these patients, about one out of ten, controlling posture, modifying activities, and avoiding pain-producing movements are more important. And remember: exercise is only one prong of the Four A program. Your confident attitude, the constructive changes in your activities, and your ability to take charge are essential. No one should expect to remain pain-free with just ten minutes of back exercise a day.

Before you recoil at the sight of so many exercises, take note that nobody is suggesting that you attempt them all. Keep in mind that this is a permissive program, and what you are offered here is a wide selection of exercises from which to choose a few that suit your needs. These are exercises for people who hate exercise — but who presumably hate back pain even more.

Certainly some exercises are harder than others, but it would be wrong to describe any as better than others.

"Better" depends entirely on your experience and your needs. What you should be looking for are at least three — or as many as six — exercises that keep your back feeling good. Don't feel guilty if you pick several of the easiest; if they work, they're right for you. And don't feel any obligation to progress from easy exercises to difficult ones. As long as those you choose are helping your back, you can stay with them indefinitely.

I have divided the exercises according to their use for each of the patterns of pain. They are grouped according to the starting position — standing, sitting, or lying down. I've separated those for pain control, mainly stretching, from those for physical conditioning. For pain control, you usually move in one direction, away from the pain. Your routines for recovery of movement and strength are more balanced.

Regardless of the exercises you choose, set aside ten minutes out of every twenty-four hours. For pain control, the time is best divided into brief periods spread over the day. For movement and strength, it's more effective to select one convenient time. Either way, make sure you exercise daily. You won't be helping yourself if you skip days and then try to make up the time in hour-long bursts of effort. In only ten minutes a day, you are unlikely to have time for more than three of the exercises on the list. Of course, you are free to increase the amount of time you work out; this is a permissive program. But to break the monotony, you might select six exercises you like and alternate them — three one day, another three the next.

Don't rush through any exercise. You're not in a race, and you'll benefit more if you take your time. Repeat the motions of each exercise as often as you think is sensible — about ten repetitions is average — or until you have filled your allotted time for the day. And don't let it get out of control. I have known many back patients, myself included, to gradually expand the exercise period to two hours or more as they gain strength. Then, when the exercises become too much of a nuisance, they simply stop. It's easier to quit altogether than to cut down to what you can reasonably handle.

Read the instructions carefully and follow them closely. In particular, make sure that your starting position is correct. This is important not only to make the exercise effective but also to avoid needless discomfort. If an exercise does cause pain, don't abandon it without considering first what kind of pain you feel.

Muscular pain may develop from the unaccustomed exercising of neglected muscles. This is no cause for alarm. If possible, put up with the discomfort or "strain pain" until the muscles stop complaining. Or, if you prefer, switch to another exercise for a day or two and then go back to the first one when those sore muscles have had a rest.

Aggravation of back pain is not dangerous or harmful in moderate doses, but it may discourage you from continuing. No pain control exercise should increase the very pain you are trying to eliminate. If the exercise intensifies your typical pain, you may be using the wrong routine for your pattern. But it's very important to separate unwanted aggravation from "centralization." The concept of centralization originated with Robin McKenzie, a physiotherapist from New Zealand. McKenzie noted that during some exercises a patient's typical pain tended to migrate toward the center of the low back and might increase. As strange as it sounds, this is a good sign; it's an indication that the exercise is having the desired pain control effect. The original pain disappears and with time the centralized pain begins to subside. The opposite is also true. If your exercises seem to push the pain farther into your buttock or down your leg, the treatment direction may be wrong. I suggest that you check with your doctor or your physiotherapist.

Common backache is mechanical pain. Mechanical pain means pain arising from wear in the physical structures in your back — the discs or joints, for example. It should respond rapidly to movement or position as you load or unload the painful structures. The effect can be like a light switch turning the pain on and off. Both the positive and negative responses are often quicker than you or your doctor might anticipate. The signs of easily controllable mechanical pain are its predictable response to exercise and its brief disappearance during particular activities. Of course, not all back pain is so straightforward, and if you can't recognize a consistent pattern, again I suggest you check with your doctor or physiotherapist.

My exercise descriptions include terms you may find unfamiliar:

Prone means lying on your stomach.

Supine means lying on your back with your legs straight.

Crook lying means lying on your back with your hips and knees bent and your feet flat on the floor.

Half-crook lying means lying on your back with one hip and knee bent and one leg straight on the floor.

For each exercise, repeat the movements about ten times, or hold the positions for five to ten seconds before relaxing slowly. The details are up to you; experiment and find the best routine. There are no wrong choices; some choices are just more effective than others.

PAIN CONTROL EXERCISES FOR PATTERN ONE

STANDING

1. Arching Backward

Exercise: Stand with your feet comfortably apart and your hands on your buttocks. Push your hips forward as you arch backward to look at the ceiling. Keep your knees as straight as possible.

Comment: This is an action you already know: it's one you use instinctively after you have been sitting for a long time. By turning it into an exercise and scheduling it throughout the day, you gain sustained pain control.

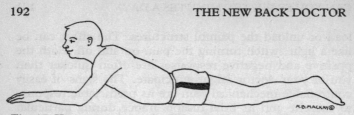

Fig. 17. You can assume the TV position on your forearms or elbows. Arch your back, but keep your hips on the floor. This is a pain control position for Pattern 1 pain.

SITTING
2. Seated Extension

Exercise: For this you need a stool or bench without a back-rest. Grip the sides of the seat with your hands to maintain balance and lean back as far as you can.

Comment: Sitting fixes the lower body and forces you to arch your back. This is one exercise you can do at work and people will hardly notice.

LYING DOWN
3. Prone Lying

Exercise: That's all there is. Just lie on your stomach and let gravity help sag your back. Any comfortable surface will do. It's the easiest ten-minutes-a-day exercise you will find.

Comment: Some patients with Pattern One pain and very stiff spines may find even this exercise too painful. Try lying over a pillow at the front of your pelvis; that reduces the arch in your back. As the pain subsides, progress by removing the pillow.

4. The TV Position

Exercise: Prop yourself on your forearms or elbows like a child watching television. Another easy exercise.

Comment: This position increases the arch in the low back and is the next exercise after prone lying.

5. *The Sloppy Push-Up*

Exercise: Lie prone with your palms on the floor just beside your shoulders. Slowly push your head and shoulders up while your hips stay down. Try to straighten your arms fully and lock your elbows. Hold your chin tucked on your chest. To increase the sag in the small of your back, breathe in before you start and breathe out at the top of the push-up.

Comment: This is the most popular extension stretching exercise for Pattern One pain control. It is the activity that most often produces centralization. If it arches your back too much, move your hands up towards your head and try again.

PAIN CONTROL EXERCISES FOR PATTERN TWO

STANDING

6. *The Standing Pelvic Tilt*

Exercise: Stand with your back against a wall and your heels about 6 inches (15 cm) from the baseboard. Tilt your pelvis by pulling in your stomach and squeezing your buttocks together gently. You should feel your back flatten against the wall. Keep your shoulders relaxed and don't hold your breath.

Comment: Once you have the knack of the standing pelvic tilt, you can do it anywhere, substituting an imaginary wall for the real one. If you can't get the knack of the standing tilt, start by trying it lying down (Exercise 10).

7. *One-Toe Touching*

Exercise: Stand with one foot on a stool or bench directly in front of you. Bend at the waist until your chest touches your raised thigh and your hands reach the toes of the raised foot. Change legs and repeat.

Comment: This is a gentle standing flexion stretch. Movement is limited by the raised knee. You may feel

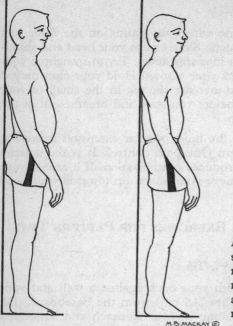

Fig. 18. The standing pelvic tilt may be difficult to master. Starting against a wall makes it easier.

M.B.MACKAY ©

some pulling in the back of the straight leg. If this helps reduce your symptoms, add extra repetitions when that leg is on the floor.

8. Two-Toe Touching

Exercise: Keep both legs relaxed but straight. Keep your feet slightly apart and your arms at your sides. Bend forward at the waist while your arms dangle in front of you. Move down slowly until your back is parallel with the floor. Don't hold this position; straighten up again as soon as you have felt a comfortable stretch.

Comment: This exercise must be done slowly. Hurling your body towards your feet in a violent ballistic action will give anyone backache. Whether you actually touch your toes isn't important; it's the movement that counts.

SITTING

9. Seated Flexion

Exercise: Sit on a chair with your legs apart, your knees bent, and your feet on the floor. Bend forward at the waist as you run your hands down the insides of your lower legs towards your ankles. Finish when your head is between your knees. Move slowly, and don't stay in the forward bent position.

Comment: How far you bend isn't significant. The idea is to feel the stretch. To make the pull more intense, straighten your knees before you try to slide your hands down to your ankles.

LYING DOWN

10. The Pelvic Tilt

Exercise: Start in the crook lying position, on your back with your knees bent. Tighten your stomach muscles and flatten the small of your back against the floor by rolling your hips forward. Raise your buttocks slightly but don't lift or push with your feet.

Comment: The pelvic tilt is not so much an exercise as a starting position for many of the flexion strengthening routines. It can, however, be an effective pain control movement for Pattern Two.

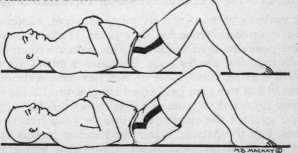

Fig. 19. The pelvic tilt is basic to most abdominal exercises and is a pain control position for Pattern 2.

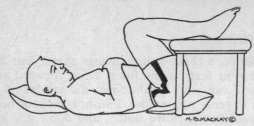

Fig. 20. The "Z"-lying is a good defensive position for both mechanical back pain and Pattern 3 leg pain. You can adjust the thickness of the pillow, the height of the stool, and the amount you bend your knees.

11. Both Knees to Chest

Exercise: Lie in the crook position and perform a pelvic tilt. Now grasp the backs of your thighs and draw your bent knees onto your chest. Pull slowly and feel the stretch before letting go.

Comment: If your arms aren't long enough to reach your legs, slip a towel behind your thighs and pull up on the ends. Pulling one leg at a time provides some hip stretch but has almost no effect on the low back or on Pattern Two pain.

PAIN CONTROL EXERCISES FOR PATTERN THREE

For patients with an acutely pinched nerve, exercise in the conventional sense has little place. However, several of the positions used in Pattern One pain are often helpful in reducing the leg pain. Exercises 3 and 4 are well suited, and Exercise 5 can sometimes have a dramatic effect. All of these are performed lying down. Eliminating gravity decreases the pressure that causes the disc to protrude against the nerve. Resting on your hands and knees, like the patient I described earlier in this book, may be beneficial. A completely different anti-gravity position that many Pattern Three patients find useful is a variation of crook lying.

LYING DOWN
12. "Z"-Lying

Exercise: Lie on your back with both knees bent and your lower legs resting on a bench, stool, or the seat of a chair. Put your head on a pillow and tuck another one under your buttocks. Move as close to the chair as possible so your knees are bent up over your abdomen and you are shaped like the letter "Z." Rest in this position as long as the leg pain is controlled.

Comment: Small adjustments to the thickness of the pillows or the height of the chair seat are often necessary to increase the comfort.

PAIN CONTROL EXERCISES FOR PATTERN FOUR

Most patients with Pattern Four symptoms — leg pain brought on by walking and relieved by rest — are helped by forward bending. The same exercises employed in Pattern Two are worthwhile here. Exercises 6, 8, and 10 are particularly effective.

Pattern Four often requires more than short-term pain control. For lasting improvement, patients with this pattern of pain need physical conditioning, notably flexion strengthening exercises.

PHYSICAL CONDITIONING IN FLEXION

Start these exercises lying on your back. The degree of difficulty can be altered by changing the arm position. The easiest variation is with the arms extended over the legs. Folding the arms over the chest makes the exercise more difficult, and holding the hands beside the ears, with the elbows out to the sides, is the most challenging. The hands are not locked behind the head because of the tendency to pull the head forward when compensating for weak abdominal muscles. Neck pain can result from flexion exercises for the low back. Keep the chin tucked against the chest and try to lift the head and upper torso as a single unit.

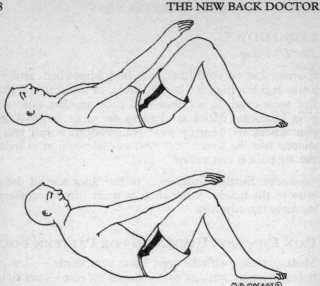

Fig. 21. The part sit-up is an excellent upper abdominal strengthening exercise. Maintain your pelvic tilt and avoid thrusting your head forward.

13. The Part Sit-Up

Exercise: Begin in a crook lying position with a pelvic tilt. Using your abdominal muscles, raise your upper body slowly until your shoulder blades clear the floor. Keep your feet down. Hold and slowly release.

Comment: When done properly, this is, in my opinion, the most effective flexion strengthening exercise. Many people, however, hook their feet under a heavy piece of furniture before they begin. That's a mistake. If your feet are restrained, the sit-up becomes a leg exercise offering little benefit for the abdomen. And don't push your chin forward to offset weak belly muscles.

Another common technical error is to stop before the shoulder blades lift. Most of the effort, and therefore most of the benefit, occurs at this point. Too little movement reduces the value of the exercise. Performing a full sit-up is also inefficient. The last thirty degrees of elevation are easily achieved and require little strength. This exercise is a sit-up with a built-in rest period.

14. The Sit-Down

Exercise: Sit and hug your knees. Without letting go, lean slowly backward until your elbows are straight. Use your arms to pull yourself up again or let go and allow your shoulders to sink to the floor.

Comment: This is a way to start if you find you have little or no strength in your abdominal muscles. Your arms provide the power. Gradually you will be able to return to the upright seated position without using your arms. The sit-down becomes the sit-up. But be patient; it takes months to develop the abdominal muscles.

15. The Oblique Sit-Up

Exercise: Adopt a crook lying position and hold a pelvic tilt. Slowly raise your head and shoulders until the shoulder blades lift. Bend slightly to one side as if you were going to reach the outside of your knee. Hold, relax, and then start again, bending to the other side.

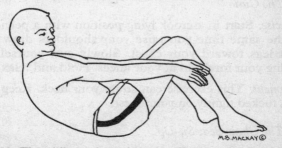

Fig. 22. The oblique sit-up is most effective when your head and shoulders face forward and the sideways movement occurs only through the trunk. This exercise strengthens the muscles on the sides of your body and helps slim your waistline.

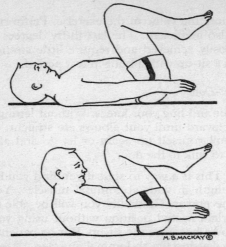

Fig. 23. The curl is an abdominal strengthening exercise. It puts you in a fetal position while lying on your back, which helps Pattern 2 or 4 pain.

Comment: Moving slightly to one side works the oblique muscles around your trunk, as well as the central muscle bands, the rectus abdominis.

16. *The Curl*

Exercise: Start in a crook lying position with a pelvic tilt. At the same time you raise your shoulders draw your bent legs toward your chest. Slowly curl yourself up, aiming your forehead at your knees. Hold and relax.

Comment: This exercise can strain your neck. Keep your chin tucked tightly on your chest.

17. *The Chair Seat Sit-Up*

Exercise: Lie on your back with your hips and knees bent and your calves on the seat of a chair. Maintain a pelvic tilt and slowly sit up until your shoulder blades clear the floor. Hold and gradually release.

Comment: Putting your legs up removes almost all the help you get from your hip muscles when you do a sit-up. This version forces you to use nothing but your abdominal muscles. It's tough. You can make it tougher by changing the position of your arms.

Other flexion strengthening exercises rely on the abdominal muscle contractions generated by lifting the legs.

18. The Cross-Arm Knee Push

Exercise: From a crook lying position and a pelvic tilt, bring one knee towards your chest and press against it with the opposite arm. Raise your head and shoulder slightly and keep your elbow straight. Hold, relax, and repeat using the other arm and leg.

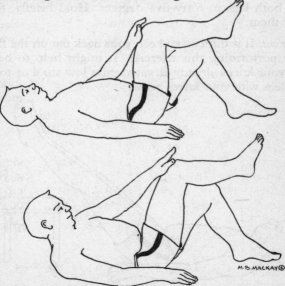

Fig. 24. While performing the cross-arm knee push, tuck your chin to avoid neck strain. Apply as much pressure as you can without moving.

Comment: This is an isometric exercise, which means there should be no movement. The tension in the muscles is created by pressure against a fixed point.

19. Single Leg Lifts

Exercise: Start in a half-crook position. Lift your straight leg to the level of your bent knee, then lower it again. Repeat, then change sides.

Comment: This exercise is easier when you bend your knee as you lift your leg. It is more difficult when you start in a supine position and lift your leg straight.

20. Double Leg Lifts

Exercise: From a supine position with a pelvic tilt, slowly raise both legs to forty-five degrees. Hold briefly, then lower them.

Comment: It is difficult to keep your back flat on the floor while performing this exercise. It might help to begin with your knees already elevated on a low stool or to lift your legs with your knees bent.

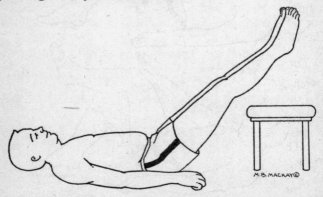

Fig. 25. Double leg raising may force you to arch your back. Start from a stool or bend your knees. It is a good lower abdominal strengthening exercise.

21. Leg Spreading

Exercise: Lie supine and hold a pelvic tilt. Bend both knees toward your chest, then straighten your legs and lower them to a forty-five degree angle with the floor. Now spread your legs apart and bring them back together.

Comment: The closer your legs are to the floor, the more difficult the exercise becomes and the greater the tendency to lose your pelvic tilt. The exercise is more demanding if you lift your legs with your knees straight. You can do the same exercise seated with your palms on the floor behind you for support. Bend your knees to your chest, straighten your legs, and spread them in midair. To make it even more interesting, try holding your arms out to the sides and balancing on your buttocks.

PHYSICAL CONDITIONING IN EXTENSION

Start these exercises lying on your stomach. Like the flexion strengthening group, you can change the difficulty of these exercises by changing your arm position. Clasping your hands behind the small of your back makes the exercise easier. Clasping your hands behind your neck is an intermediate position, and extending your arms over your head adds the most difficulty. To avoid neck pain, keep your chin tucked.

22. Trunk Extension

Exercise: Lie prone. Slowly raise your head and chest until they clear the floor.

Comment: Whether you hold the position or do repetitions is your choice. Whatever works best for you is correct. This exercise is more difficult than it seems, so start slowly.

23. Trunk and Leg Extension

Exercise: Lie prone. Tuck your chin and raise your head and upper body at the same time you lift both legs with the knees bent until your thighs leave the floor.

Comment: To do this exercise properly requires strong back muscles. Start slowly, with your hands behind the small of your back. The difficulty increases if you keep your legs straight and lift from your hips.

24. Assisted Extension

Exercise: Lie prone on a table or firm mattress with your legs and hips on the surface and your body from the waist up hanging over the edge. With someone or something holding your legs down, raise your upper body to the horizontal, so your back is in a straight line.

Comment: In my opinion, this is the best of the extension strengthening exercises. It develops the paraspinal muscles without forcing the back into a markedly extended position. And lifting the weight of your torso ten times can be a daunting task. Unlike the part sit-up, you need help with the assisted extension. Holding your feet down in this extension exercise keeps you from landing on your head.

A few extension strengthening exercises develop the back muscles by extending the hips or arms or both because the muscles along the spine contract whenever the limbs are moved.

25. Hip Extension

Exercise: While lying prone, bend one knee and lift your thigh off the floor.

Comment: Hold the position or repeat the movement. The lift is more difficult if you keep the leg straight. Moving your hip backward strengthens both muscles along the spine and in the buttock.

26. Arm Extension

Exercise: Lie on your stomach with your arms straight out on the floor above your head. Lift one arm off the floor, hold it, then lower it.

Comment: This is an easy strengthening exercise. For someone with weak back muscles, it may be a place to start, but it's only a small first step. The exercise can be made somewhat more strenuous by lifting one arm and the opposite leg at the same time.

LEG-STRENGTHENING EXERCISES

27. *The Half-Knee Bend*

Exercise: Stand erect with your hands on your hips. Slowly bend your knees, keeping your feet flat on the floor. Stop when your knees are bent between forty-five and sixty degrees, and come back up.

Comment: For maximum benefit, bend and straighten slowly. When you descend quickly, you are relying on gravity instead of your thigh muscles. I choose half-bends rather than deep knee bends to reduce complaints of knee pain and to minimize the bouncing movement some people use to complete the exercise.

28. *The Imaginary Chair*

Exercise: Stand with your back pressed against a smooth wall and your heels about 12 inches (30 cm) in front of the baseboard. Slide your body down slowly until you are positioned as if you were seated in a chair, with your thighs parallel to the floor. Don't move your feet forward; keep them directly under your knees. Hold this position as long as you can. Don't press with your hands on the tops of your knees. That makes the exercise easier, and that's cheating.

Comment: Most people who have never tried the Imaginary Chair find it hard to hold for thirty seconds. Don't despair; just do what you can, relax, and repeat. After some days or weeks, you will work your way up to a respectable period. Three minutes is considered an achievement by most fit people; if you last more than five minutes, you are ready for the Olympics.

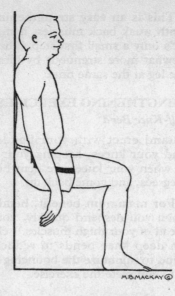

Fig. 26. The imaginary chair is a challenging thigh strengthening exercise. Press your back against the wall to hold your position.

M.B.MACKAY ©

One final word on exercise. Important though it is, your routine of back exercise is not the entire long-term solution to your back problem. It would be unrealistic to expect ten minutes of daily exercise to provide you with control of your symptoms throughout the other twenty-three hours and fifty minutes. Exercise is just one part of a control program that must also include techniques for protecting your back during all your activities of daily living. Although the importance of this aspect of your program may not be as obvious as the importance of exercise, it is equally significant.

But before we move on to the business of long-term control of your back, we must face the immediate problem of coping with your next acute attack.

12 *Be Ready for That Next Attack*

Nothing will boost your morale and build your self-confidence faster than knowing how to cope with a sudden attack of back pain. As you have probably discovered the hard way, an acute attack can be triggered by the most trivial, routine action — reaching up to a shelf, opening a window, or bending over to put on your shoes. In fact, the action may be so familiar that you cannot even identify it as the movement that triggered your attack. It is important to realize that the triggering incident does not damage your back; it simply activates the source of your pain. In any case, you may find it impossible to avoid all actions and situations that are potential "triggers." The solution, instead, is to be so well informed and prepared that you can deal calmly with an attack from the moment it begins. In that frame of mind, you can avoid the panic that causes your system to tighten up and aggravate your condition.

Typically, an attack is signaled by a sudden stab of pain followed rapidly by a muscle spasm. After that, the two may interact repeatedly. The strategy, then, is to take protective action so promptly that the initial pain is eased and the spasm never occurs.

Basic Defense Positions

At the first sign of an attack, use the pain control maneuver you have found most effective. This may mean lying on your stomach, resting on your elbows, or curling up in a fetal position, either on your back or on one side: knees bent up to your chest and chin tucked well down. Your goals are to get out of the upright position so that gravity is no longer creating a load on your spine and to tilt your pelvis in one direction or the other to change the curve in your low back and eliminate extra stress. No one position works for everyone. In the beginning, at least, your own routine is the result of trial and error. Just remember, you can't damage your spine by experimenting.

My favorite position was described in the last chapter as a pain control exercise for Pattern Three (Exercise 12). I don't have a pinched nerve and my pain is purely mechanical Pattern One, but the position works for me, so I use it. As quickly as I can, I lie down with pillows under my head and buttocks and my legs up on a chair seat. Once safe in this position, I stay free of pain. It may not be the "correct" solution for my particular pain pattern, but I don't care because it makes me feel better.

Of course, pillows and chairs may not be easy to find in the middle of the mall, so it's a good idea to develop alternative strategies. I get rapid relief from the sloppy push-up (Exercise 5). You may feel silly, but with a little ingenuity you can do it almost anywhere. Another position I use often involves hugging one knee as tightly to my chest as I can. Preferably, this is done lying down, but if you can't lie down, you can sit with your back in a corner to provide support. A pillow or lumbar roll in the small of the back aids comfort. The lumbar roll is a five-inch (13 cm) diameter firm foam roll. It's usually about 12 inches (30.5 cm) long and so can be carried easily. Some back pain sufferers consider it the height of fashion.

The squat is another good position to assume. I use it a lot myself, especially if I am taking a short break between stints in the operating room. It's a helpful way to reduce the tension on the spine for a few minutes and thereby ward off an attack. The squat has one drawback, though: once you're into it, you may find you need somebody to help you stand up again. If you're not an experienced squatter, squat with your back to a wall; otherwise, you may tip over. In fact, you can use the wall as a means of assuming the position. Stand with your back against the wall, then bend your knees and slide down until you have reached a full squat.

All these alternatives achieve the same basic effects: they unload the spine, alter the curve in the low back, and provide rapid pain control.

If you have an attack when your choice of positions is limited by practical or social considerations, you may have to compromise a little.

At your desk in the office, for instance, try drawing one leg up to your chest and resting the heel of that foot on the seat of your chair. If you have a tilting chair, you may be able to tilt back and push one foot or both against the edge of your desk — a sort of White Collar Fetal Position. If you have a door on your office and a carpet on the floor, it's the perfect place for ten sloppy push-ups or a few minutes of lying on your stomach, or whatever works best for you. I know one executive whose secretary kept track of the number of times a day he quietly closed the door to his office. When the frequency dropped and his back pain increased, she scheduled the pain control periods for him.

If you are behind the wheel of your car when your back starts to tighten up, you can consider several options, depending upon the circumstances. If you are cruising on the highway or driving anywhere in a car without a clutch, you can probably manage to bend your left leg until your left foot is near the seat. If you are able to pull off the road and stop, you may be able to get out and squat beside the car until the attack begins to subside. Keep a small pillow or lumbar roll handy. Slip it behind the small of your back before you drive off. I get the best relief by removing the lumbar roll in half an hour or so. Putting it in and taking it out changes the curve in my low back and eliminates constant pressure on the sore spots.

On an aircraft, you can use your seat belt to good advantage: cinch it tightly to hold yourself well back in the seat after rolling an airline pillow behind your lower back, and support your feet on a piece of hand luggage, so that your knees are higher than your hips. Always choose an aisle seat so you can stand and stretch frequently. Don't be self-conscious; just reach up toward the overhead compartment and pretend to check your luggage, or walk up to the front of the plane to give the captain some advice.

If an attack occurs when you are standing and you can't get off your feet, try arching backward (Exercise 1) or a pelvic tilt (Exercise 6) and, if possible, put one foot up on a rail or curb or anything else that's handy. These maneuvers relax or stretch the spinal muscles and restore the normal amount of curve to the low back. A rapid change in posture is the next best thing to lying down.

If you have found, during a previous attack, that some particular position provides you with better pain relief, use it. Don't feel bound by the suggestions you see here. They are the positions that help most people, but you may be different. It's up to you to find the best way of coping with your back pain.

Your strategy should be defensive. This is not the best time to begin experimenting with new gimmicks or the latest back aid you just saw on T.V. There is no danger, no chance of harming your spine, but there is also little chance of success. Any extra discomfort may frighten you and the fear can aggravate the intensity of your attack. Your best bet is to rely on simple methods of posture correction, gentle stretches away from the pain, anti-gravity positions, and the appropriate pain control exercise.

If you're unlucky enough to have a cold coming on while your back is sore, try to remember this four-line jingle:

> *To save your back*
> *When you cough or sneeze*
> *Unload your spine*
> *As you bend your knees.*

Even the best preventive measures are not foolproof. Sometimes an attack will occur and persist despite your best efforts. When that happens, try to keep one point in mind: no attack is a total setback. The exercises you have done and the good postural habits you have assumed will count for something sooner or later. Even if the new attack produces pain that's as bad as ever, you will likely recover sooner than you did from previous episodes.

Be Patient — Time Is on Your Side

Once you have done all you can to ward off the attack, you have no option but to wait until the pain subsides. Most acute episodes end quickly, within days or weeks. Nearly ninety percent of attacks disappear within two months. That's little consolation on Day One, but then I'm not advising you just to lie there and take it. In fact, I'm not telling you to lie down at all. Short periods of rest are desirable. There is no substitute for rest in a recumbent position to remove the compressive effect of gravity, but that doesn't mean going to bed for a week. There is no single correct surface on which you must lie. Some people prefer the floor, others a firm mattress, and still others a stiffly padded chair. They are all fine, just as long as you are comfortable and your back has a chance to relax in the position best suited to relieve your pain. Bed rest on a poor mattress or sitting in an overstuffed chair can create more back pain than walking to the corner store. Stay as active as you can, and keep in mind that your pain is not a signal of irreversible damage. In the mechanical back attack, hurt does not mean harm.

Your rate of recovery depends upon the amount of wear in your spine and the pattern of your pain; Pattern Two usually gets better faster than Pattern One. It also reflects your skill at pain control and your ability to temporarily adjust your lifestyle. Make it a rule to discontinue all activities that aggravate the pain until the worst part of the attack is over. This temporary ban on certain activities is not to prevent you from harming yourself — that wouldn't happen — but to prevent you from becoming discouraged by the frequent recurrence of your pain. Sometimes people who practice active pain control forget how important it is to avoid painful situations at the same time. As a result, they become so disenchanted with the whole program that they simply give up. I hope you won't make that mistake. You will find there are substitute activities and different ways of doing the same thing that will keep you productive even during the height of the attack. Be creative.

There is no harm in taking a pain-reliever, but I don't recommend narcotics. In the proper treatment of back pain, there is little place for the use of such drugs. If narcotics are used regularly, we face the specter of addiction. Stay with over-the-counter medications. If your doctor prescribes some stronger medicine, use it only as directed. And don't lose sight of the fact that most back pain is a mechanical problem, best treated by mechanical means, the sort of postures and exercises I have described.

Try counter-irritants if you wish. The choice is entirely yours. If a cold pack or a heating pad helps relieve your pain, indulge yourself. A hot bath and a hot toddy can work wonders.

Anti-inflammatory drugs are no substitutes for good back care and physical activity. Their effects are unpredictable. If you are among those who have success with them, use them. But don't build your personal recovery program around them.

Back braces and corsets may be useful to people whose jobs or other obligations require them to carry on. The best device of this kind, in my opinion, is a lightweight, adjustable, easily removable support belt. Anyone can obtain considerable comfort from such appliances, but they should be used only as a temporary means of relief. An effective support garment doesn't help your back directly, but it acts as a reminder to avoid improper body mechanics and has a reassuring effect that is beneficial even to people whose muscles are strong.

Once again I must emphasize that there are no "bests" or absolutes for anyone. There are just two basic principles to remember:

1. Use whatever pain control technique works best for you. Do it often.
2. For as long as the severe attack persists, avoid the activities that trigger the pain. It's a temporary restriction.

Once your acute attack has subsided — and every acute attack does subside — you will want to get on with the task of maintaining long-term control and going about the business of preventing an acute episode from ever happening again.

13 *Living with Your Back*

It would be possible to list dozens of rules for avoiding backache during your activities of daily living — your ADL — but, as you realize by now, I'm not inclined toward rule-making, either for my readers or for my back patients. I have always found it more practical to stress the right attitude by setting out general principles and then illustrating them with examples.

First, three essentials, in principle:

1. Hold your low back in a neutral curve, or as close to it as circumstances allow, throughout virtually every activity. Too much slump or too much arch means backache.

2. When lifting objects, let your legs do some of the work by squatting or knee-bending. Your back is not a crane.

3. Find ways to assist your spine by improving the mechanical advantage. For example, don't pick up a heavy object at arm's length if you can hug it against your body.

Now let's see how these principles can be applied to various activities.

Night Rest

You can maintain your correct back posture by lying on your back with a small pillow under your head and your legs kept in a moderate crook position. As you may have discovered, solid foam pillows are hard on your neck, so if you have neck pain along with back trouble, use a pillow filled with feathers, down, soft foam chips, or the new synthetic fillers. Support your knees with a large pillow or two, perhaps wrapped in a sheet or blanket. Wrapping the pillows keeps them in place as you sleep. A thick bolster works well. One alternative: raise your lower legs with one or two seat cushions — if you can find a way of keeping them in place all night. If you prefer to sleep on your side, curl into a ball and place a pillow between your knees to prevent your pelvis from rotating. Many people find it more comfortable to draw up only the top leg. Whichever position you use, keep the pillow between your thighs.

One of the best ideas I know to promote a comfortable night's sleep, in spite of a sore back, is to use a rolled towel around your waist. When you lie down, your lower spine is suspended between your chest and your hips, like a clothesline between two poles. No matter what position you adopt as you sleep, your back sags, putting extra pressure on areas that may cause pain. Supporting your back with a rolled towel keeps it in line and evens the load. The thickness of the roll depends upon the gap between your waist and hips. Experiment until you find the size that's right for you; not too thick, not too thin. I call this my Michelin technique because with a large roll belted or pinned around your waist, you will look like their trademark tire-man. You may feel a little foolish, but you will be amazed how well you sleep. Incidentally, the same approach is great for neck pain. A rolled towel along the bottom of the pillow inside the pillowcase fills the space between your head and shoulder. It's an inexpensive way to eliminate night-time neck pain.

Sleeping on your stomach can lead to morning backache. Or you may find it is the only way to get comfortable. It depends upon your pattern of pain and your personal preference. There is no right answer. Doctors used to insist that sleeping on the stomach was "bad" for the back. People who found it the only relaxing way to sleep were told to use some other (uncomfortable) position. That makes no sense. No posture can harm your spine. If sleeping on your stomach feels good, do it. In this case, you are the best judge of what is best for you.

Day Rest

Here are three positions favored by most back patients, especially when recovering from a pain attack.

Position 1: For reading or watching television while lying down, lie on the floor on your back with your legs in a crook position. Place a fairly thick pillow under your head and a slim pillow under your buttocks to keep a gentle curve in your back. If the floor feels too hard, use a chaise longe cushion, or similar long pad, as a mattress.

Position 2: Use a large pillow under your head and shoulders and another one under your buttocks. Rest your legs on a chair seat or padded table. Of course, you recognize this as Exercise 12, my favorite defensive position. I am sure that this position has saved me from a severe attack of back pain on at least one occasion. I was carrying a heavy armload of firewood into the house when I lost my footing on the doorstep. In an effort to keep from falling, I twisted my back and felt something happen — I'm sure you know the feeling.

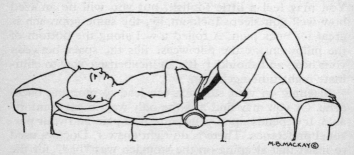

M.B.MACKAY©

Fig. 27. Resting positions unload the low back by eliminating gravity and restoring a neutral lordosis. The lumbar support will be effective only on a firm surface.

Fortunately, it was a Sunday afternoon and there was a good football game on television, and so I took to the living room floor, watched the game, and remained in this position for several hours. The attack I anticipated never developed.

Position 3: Lying prone and resting on your forearms is a position that many people find reduces back pain. This posture is particularly helpful in Pattern One. If you lie on your stomach long enough, you may feel a different sort of back pain so it's a good idea to change positions every so often. No posture, no matter how perfect, should be held all day.

Sitting

Most people don't realize that sitting is hard on your back. As you may recall from my comments in Chapter Three, there is a greater load on the discs in your spine when you are in a sitting position, especially if you are bending forward, than when you are standing erect. This is one reason why many people with desk jobs complain of back pain.

Start with a comfortable chair — well padded but not overstuffed. It should have a firm back that slopes backward about ten degrees and a seat that supports your thighs slightly above the level of your hips. Rocking chairs are great, but they do make desk work difficult.

If you are concerned about choosing an office or work chair, your best choice is a tilter that also locks upright. With it, you can either lock it to gain support for your lumbar spine or release it to allow you to tilt back and relax. Arm rests give you the opportunity to raise your upper body and briefly take the load off your lower back. The seat should be wide enough to allow you to shift your weight. Also, make sure it treats your legs right: the front of the seat shouldn't cut into the backs of your thighs. A footrest on the chair or a footstool nearby will help if your legs can't reach the floor easily. Whatever

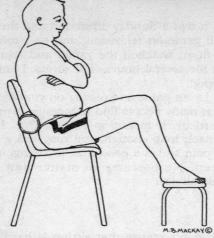

Fig. 28. Prolonged sitting is particularly uncomfortable for patients with Pattern 1 pain. Restoring a normal curve to the low back reduces the discomfort. Even a good sitting posture may become uncomfortable, so change your position frequently.

arrangement you have, change your position frequently to share the load between the discs and joints.

If most of your day is spent sitting, then proper sitting posture must be a major concern. Sitting reduces the normal low back curve and increases the strain on the front of the spine. Restoring a balanced curve almost always means arching the low back. The regular use of a lumbar support — I prefer the 5-inch (13 cm) firm foam lumbar roll — can be the most important thing you do to prevent future backache.

Here are three solutions to the problem of sitting with a bad back.

Position 1: Slide your buttocks to the back of a firm chair. Lean forward slightly and place the lumbar roll behind your back at about belt level. The fine adjustments are up to you. Bend back just enough to reduce your discomfort. If your legs are too short to rest on the floor, use a footstool.

Position 2: Sit on the floor with your back against a wall and hug your knees.

Position 3: Hunker down. Variations on the squat are used throughout the world, with great versatility and little backache. If you aren't used to squatting, however, and you are a bit older, you may find it hard on the knees. Compromise by going down on one knee with the other foot flat on the floor. Try to squat in any situation where you might otherwise kneel fully or bend at the waist. The squat is ideal for tending your garden, hobnobbing with small children, or socializing at informal parties where some guests sprawl on the floor.

I'm sure you get the idea. Each of these positions requires you to adjust the curve in your low back and reduces the excessive strain of slumping forward when you sit. For most of us in North America, Position 1 is the most practical, but go ahead — invent your own.

One of the best opportunities for planning your sitting to protect your back arises every time you travel on an airplane. Remember the tricks I outlined in the last chapter: a pillow for lumbar support, hand luggage for a footstool, the seat belt to keep you from slipping forward, and an aisle seat so you can stand and stretch. Even long flights should present no problems if you follow these simple suggestions. The same principles will allow you to sit anywhere for as long as you require.

Home Duties — Sitting

Again, observe the principles of a neutral curve and you can't go far wrong. In the kitchen, keep utensils within easy reach. Where a low chair won't do, use a high stool with a step or rung for your feet. When reading, support your arms on a table or desk. Keep a lumbar roll handy. With that simple addition for low back support, the straight-backed kitchen chair may become the most comfortable chair in the house.

Home Duties — Standing

Never stand flat-footed if you can put one foot up on a stool or low shelf — the posture drinkers assume at a stand-up bar. Saloon keepers discovered the comfort of this position long before doctors understood the theory behind it, and there's no reason why you can't enjoy its advantages in your own home. It's just another way of maintaining a balanced lumbar curve.

During activities that may aggravate your pain — bending into low cupboards, cleaning overhead shelves — rotate your activities to avoid prolonged strain. Rest often, if only for a few minutes each time.

Sweeping the floor, vacuuming a carpet, and raking the leaves can all cause pain by requiring you to sustain a forward bent posture. The proper way to carry out these tasks is to use your legs, lunging like a fencer while keeping your back as upright and relaxed as possible. It may sound silly, but with practice it can be done so easily that nobody will notice, and your back will feel so much better.

Work Surfaces

For most people with back trouble, the ideal height for a work surface, such as a desk, counter, or table top, is 2 inches (5 cm) below the elbow. Since most work surfaces are non-adjustable, you should try to overcome any discrepancy by providing an item of the right height for sitting or standing, such as a stool to sit on if the surface is too low for standing comfortably. Also, keep in mind that a work surface of ideal height ceases to be ideal if you are working on an object that is tall or bulky. For example, if you try to repair a chair on top of a work bench, the operation may be too high for comfort.

Office Duties

You can do your back a great favor with a device as simple as a fat telephone directory placed under your feet while you're seated at your desk. Shift around often. Pull open a low desk drawer and use it for a footstool while you chat with a visitor or talk on the phone. Use a lumbar support and get up frequently and walk. If you're the boss, put your feet up on the desk.

Lifting

There is no single right way to lift an object. The right way in a given situation will depend upon the size and weight of the load and the conditions under which it is to be lifted, such as the access you have to it. The three basic principles are:

1. Take advantage of mechanical leverage by keeping the burden as close as possible to your body.
2. Do as much of the lifting and turning as you can with leg muscles rather than back muscles.
3. Keep your back erect and balanced. This is not the same as making it ramrod straight; some lifts require you to tilt your upper body forward, in which case you should let your hips do part of the bending while you hold that lumbar curve.

Body weight, momentum, and even gravity can be used to your advantage. The method you choose may combine these principles and forces in various ways. To lift a heavy carton from the floor, for instance, I would crouch close to it, hug it to my chest, and then rise by straightening my legs. This style of lift is good for my back, but it does place quite a strain on my knees. To lug a heavy tool chest from a high shelf and move it across the room, I would rely on gravity, momentum, and my own agility, pulling the box off the shelf and using gravity to create a momentum with which I would spin on the balls of my feet so as to move in the desired direction and carry the box, all in one continuous motion. This is one example of many lifting situations where you may be inclined to rotate your spine — a motion that is uncomfortable for any sore back. When you have to turn while lifting, avoid spinal rotation by turning your feet instead. The best lift is whatever you find, in the circumstances, to be safe, comfortable, and effective. The idea is to plan ahead. Work out the lift in your mind before you work out your muscles in the lift.

The most hazardous lifts are the ones for which you are unprepared. For example, you and a companion may be carrying a heavy chest of drawers up a staircase when he stumbles, unexpectedly shifting the whole load to you. This leaves you no time to brace yourself and protect your spine. Before you get into a situation like that, discuss the lift until you both agree on how you will provide yourselves with maximum protection in the event of a mishap. Then make sure you adopt a lifting technique that gives you maximum mechanical advantage. Use these precautions even for lifting tasks that don't seem particularly onerous.

The most difficult lift — even when you are prepared for it — is one where a heavy object must be raised at arm's length and then hoisted over a sash or barrier. One familiar example is the problem of removing an outboard motor from the trunk of a car. Another is the task of lifting a child out of a high-sided crib or playpen.

The solution is to avoid lifting from a distance and to deal with the barrier by minimizing its effect on your task. When reaching for the outboard motor, for instance, put one foot either on the bumper or, better still, right inside the car trunk. This places your body as close as possible to the burden before the lift begins. In the nursery, let the side of the crib down — if it's that kind of design — and then bend your knees as much as necessary to clasp the child close to your chest. You can save some strain if you teach the child to come to you and stand up to be lifted.

No matter how shrewd you are about sparing your back, there will be times when you simply can't avoid using and perhaps overloading those discs and joints. And that is exactly why those conditioning exercises are so important: they provide you with that reserve in your "back account" so that those unavoidable "withdrawals" can be made without needless pain.

Sexual Intercourse

Like the time-honored headache at bedtime, a back-ache can become a convenient excuse for avoiding sexual encounters. Because no one can prove you don't have back pain, your excuse for abstinence cannot be challenged successfully. Often, however, sexual frustration and upset marriages are the by-products of genuine back trouble because one partner is fearful of triggering an attack of pain. Your back problem needn't deprive you of intercourse if you protect yourself from pain in two ways: as a long-term measure, begin at once on a regular routine of physical conditioning for your trunk muscles. What better incentive could you have for getting rid of those "love handles"? And meanwhile, make an arrangement with your partner that allows you to assume the positions least likely to give you back pain.

When the woman has back pain made worse by bending forward, she may prefer to be on the bottom, in the missionary position. She may find it comfortable on her hands and knees, allowing rear entry without a great deal of movement on her part. Lying face down with her legs slightly bent is another variation that allows intercourse without much spinal flexion.

When the man has Pattern One pain, he will also find the missionary position satisfactory. He may appreciate lying on his back while his partner straddles his pelvis. One position to avoid is standing while his partner wraps her legs around his body. It's athletic and macho, but it makes your back hurt.

If the woman has Pattern Two pain, the man can help her be comfortable if he lies on his back in a crook position and allows her to straddle his pelvis and then lean forward so that her torso is horizontal and her face is close to his. She rests her elbows above or beside his shoulders to support some of her body weight. In this position, as long as her trunk is well forward, she avoids arching either her low back or her neck.

She may find more comfort if she sits astride her partner while facing his feet. In this case, she does not bend her torso forward into a horizontal position but remains leaning forward at an angle of about forty-five degrees.

Reduced back pain for both partners is provided by a variation of the classic "spoon" position. With the couple both lying on the same side and facing in the same direction, as though she was seated on his lap, the woman parts her knees enough for the man to place his knees between her thighs and gain entry.

Both partners can also minimize pain in their low backs and necks by adopting a face-to-face position while lying on their sides. For instance, the man may lie on his right side while the woman lies facing him on her left. He raises his body long enough to allow her to slip her left leg under his body and her right leg over him. Now they come together until she is, in effect, hugging his waist with her thighs. He can now achieve good stability yet free movement by placing his palms on her buttocks while she entwines her arms around his neck. Some couples find it easier to achieve this position by starting out in the position that is commonly regarded as the basic one for intercourse: that is, with the man on top of the woman. The woman raises her legs until they are wrapped around his waist. The couple then turn onto their sides.

If you have not tried the positions described here, you may find that a certain amount of experimentation is necessary before you can achieve comfort and satisfaction. If you are the one with the back problem, your partner must be patient and understanding, and you should conduct yourself in such a way as to encourage that attitude. Prolonged gentle foreplay, oral sex, and frank conversation can heighten sexual comfort and gratification without adding stress to the spine. You will find that the extra effort required of both of you will be well worthwhile; it can enhance your sex life, improve your marriage, and make your back feel better.

Pregnancy

The effect of pregnancy on back problems is a common concern. I am frequently consulted by women who want to become pregnant but are fearful of stirring up their chronic back pain. Naturally, they wonder how great the risks are and what to do to reduce them. Although backache is common, pregnancy does not guarantee back pain. I have seen cases where women with a history of chronic back trouble have gone through an entire pregnancy without so much as a twinge of back pain. On the other hand, many women have their first experience with back pain while carrying their firstborn.

I don't believe back pain should be a reason for avoiding pregnancy. Yet I see many women who tell me that they have been advised by their doctors not to start a family because of their bad back. My advice is, if you want to become pregnant, don't let your back pain stop you. If you are planning a family, you would be well advised to condition yourself through back exercises for several months in advance until you achieve the control that minimizes the likelihood of back pain.

If back pain is going to occur during pregnancy, it usually shows up in the second trimester, the middle three months, or when the full term is almost completed. Back pain associated with pregnancy is usually the product of altered body mechanics. A shift in the mother's center of gravity produces a distinctive walk and a change in the curve of the low back. Hormones designed to assist normal childbirth relax ligaments at the base of the spine and the back of the pelvis. The growth of the fetus stretches the abdominal muscles; breast enlargement strains the upper back. These changes underline once again the importance of good posture, good back care, and good physical condition before pregnancy begins.

If you attend a prenatal program, you will probably notice the similarity between the type of exercise prescribed there and the exercise program outlined in this book. The reason is that good prenatal care, like good back care, requires protection of the back and control of the abdominal muscles. Obviously, your established exercise program will need to be modified during pregnancy, but the guidelines are the same.

Some things change, of course. Those high-heeled shoes that don't necessarily cause you back pain at other times may cause trouble during pregnancy. You will need more rest, and using your usual pain-relieving positions may no longer be possible. But understanding the reasons for your pain and planning alternative pain control measures can keep you free to enjoy your pregnancy.

One problem many women overlook is the high incidence of back pain during new motherhood. Many women succeed in avoiding back pain throughout their pregnancy, only to succumb during the first weeks after the baby is born. This is a time when the new mother is faced with many unaccustomed tasks. Consequently, she is especially vulnerable during the repetitive bending and lifting involved in nursing, bathing, and dressing the baby and in handling extra laundry.

These activities take place at the very time when the mother's abdomen is still in poor condition from the effects of pregnancy and she has not yet had time to regain good muscle tone.

If you find yourself in this situation, I suggest that you pay special attention to the techniques you use in your daily tasks, so as to give your back every reasonable protection. You should also embark on a new program of exercises as soon as your doctor gives permission.

A baby carrier, worn either over the chest or on the back, is a useful way of avoiding unnecessary stress on the lower spine. The value of this device is mainly that it keeps the weight of the baby close to your body while avoiding the additional strain of lifting the baby with your arms.

Yoga

The relaxation techniques taught in yoga can benefit people with common backache at any time, even during an attack, since this discipline helps to prevent or combat muscle spasm.

Some yoga exercises are also recommended; as you may have noticed, several of the exercises described in Chapter 11 are similar to yoga exercises, and if you prefer the latter, there is no reason why you should not use them. Although they are not as specific as the pain control techniques I have described, if they reduce your pain, go ahead. Be sure to distinguish between yoga's flexion or forward-bending exercises and its extension or backward-bending ones. As with any exercise program, pick the ones that suit your needs. Our general guidelines still apply: avoid exercises that produce or expand your typical pain, but if it feels good, do it.

Sports

People with back problems sometimes avoid taking part in sports, often on the advice of their doctors. In doing so, they deprive themselves unnecessarily of healthy recreation and the pleasure of friendly competition.

Some sports, of course, are a little too vigorous for the average back pain sufferer. If you experience frequent attacks, you're unlikely to spend weekends skydiving, hang-gliding, boxing, or engaging in such field sports as pole-vaulting, shot-put, or discus. It's not that they will harm your spine, they won't; it's just that the amount of pain they will probably produce is too high a price to pay.

But that still leaves several dozen possibilities open, and if you are an otherwise healthy person with a liking for athletics, I see no reason why common backache should keep you on the sidelines. Every sport presents some degree of hazard for the participant, whether or not he or she has back problems. You can break a finger playing Ping-Pong or a thumbnail digging for clams. The trick is to understand the risks presented by the sport of your choice and conduct yourself accordingly.

I want to make it clear that I'm talking about the stresses that occur in each sport when it is played without serious mishaps. I can't help you decide whether you will find a weekend on the ski slopes worth the risk of an abrupt collision with a tree trunk or, for that matter, engulfment by an avalanche. Here we are considering only the effect on your back of the normal actions necessary in each sport.

Three forms of strain may be imposed on your spine: weight-loading, rotation, and postural strain. Weight can cause problems when an unaccustomed load compresses your discs and forces your facet joints to rub painfully together. Rotation places strain on your discs, which do not readily tolerate the twisting that pulls at the fibers of their outer shells. Postural strain hurts because it places your spine in an extreme position, robbing it of its normal flexibility. In that position, your back can suffer more pain from any blow.

Here is my estimate of how various recreational sports deserve to be rated in terms of these factors. Some sports are listed in more than one category. Before we begin, let me emphasize again that my list gives information to help you participate intelligently, not reasons to avoid a particular sport.

Weight-loading sports

Weight-lifting, an obvious candidate here, creates heavy strain on a bad back. Unless you are an experienced competitor, you might be wise to pass up this one. More tolerable weight-loading entries are curling, bowling, scuba-diving, jogging, horseback riding, motorbiking, hunting, and fishing.

Jogging may not seem like a weight-loading sport, but the repetitive impact on the shock-absorbing discs with each stride has the same effect. Trunk-strengthening exercises should be part of a complete jogging routine.

The hazards for hunters and fishermen are the heavy game, heavy fish, and heavy equipment, such as canoes and outboard motors, that need toting.

Rotation-causing sports
Squash is probably the most vigorous of these, with racketball a close second and tennis a distant third. Golf, though less lively than the racket sports, imposes a rotational force on your spine. Avid golfers with back pain may find it better to shorten each game or modify their swing. Soccer involves a lesser element of spinal rotation. Rotation isn't a serious factor in skiing, unless you ski incorrectly. Good skiers turn their legs, not their spines, and they seldom have back problems from rotational action. Baseball (including softball or fastball) could be considered rotational because of the motion involved in batting, but you are only at bat three or four times in a typical game, and the risk of back pain is therefore much less than in, say, golf.

Sports that create postural strain
Hockey is guilty of making you arch your back as you hold that stick against the ice. The three favorite net sports — tennis, badminton, and volleyball — all induce arching, at least while you're serving. Basketball, baseball, rowing, canoeing, skiing, archery, scuba-diving, and certain swimming styles, especially the breast stroke, all impose postural strain that can lead to back pain.

Cycling demands sustained flexion, but the postural strain is offset by the weight transfer from your arms to the handlebars.

Your basic strategy in picking a suitable sport should be to understand the pain-producing movements in each case and to compare them to your own pattern of pain. Where feasible, you should modify your actions or techniques to minimize the discomfort. If you're a golfer, don't lug a bagful of clubs around; recruit a caddy or use a cart. On the tennis court, modify that service to reduce the arch in your back. As a jogger, wear the proper shoes, jog on resilient surfaces whenever you can, and do your trunk-strengthening exercises. For some sports, a back brace may give you temporary comfort.

Above all, remember that, apart from the trauma of an accident — which, after all, can happen anywhere to anybody — even the most vigorous sports activities won't harm your back; they may simply make it hurt for a few days. As we've learned repeatedly throughout this book, hurt is not the same as harm, and the trade-off will be worth it to you, in immediate pleasure and in feeling like a normal person instead of a semi-invalid.

Whatever sport you choose, keep in mind that the general fitness it provides is no substitute for those special ten-minute sessions of daily exercise you need.

Your personal program of conservative back management will succeed only if you combine its four essential elements: a positive outlook, proper activities of daily living, appropriate pain control exercise, and perhaps most important of all, the attitude of a person who has taken charge of his or her back problem.

That last point was demonstrated to me again when a forty-year-old firefighter — I'll call him Mark — came to see me with disabling back pain. I assessed his problem as a Pattern One-Two combination, pain on movement both forward and backward, with enough muscle spasm to prevent him from standing straight. I saw him after he had visited a number of other doctors, after he had been off work for almost a year, after he had been told he could not return to his regular duties, and after the possibility of surgery had been raised.

Mark wanted to go back to being a firefighter but he needed help. I explained the source of his pain and stressed his ability to solve his own problem. Because of the duration and severity of his symptoms and before considering an operation, I recommended a program of supervised active rehabilitation.

Three months later, Mark returned for his second appointment with a tale of frustration. He had been denied coverage for the treatment program and had not received the supervised therapy. He had not been allowed to return to active duty but instead had been assigned to a desk job where he sat all day. Sitting actually increased his Pattern One pain. Mark was determined to return to his old job, and after his visit with me, he was convinced that it could be done.

Based on information from my books, he created his own exercise routine to control his pain. He enroled in and passed a retraining course to sharpen his firefighting skills. The third time Mark appeared in my clinic, now smartly dressed in his uniform, his back still hurt but all he needed was medical clearance to return to full duty. I gave it without hesitation.

This man had every reason to fail. He succeeded because he took responsibility for his own recovery. Mark's lesson is a simple one. Take charge of your own back. Nothing and no one can do it as well as you can.

14 *You Are Not Alone*

I hope you have recognized yourself and your symptoms repeatedly in this book. If so, you will have come to realize that as a victim of common backache, you have problems that are not unique. Millions of others suffer the same pain as yours and harbor the same concerns and fears about future attacks. I hope you prove to be one of the many who find it possible to benefit from the simple advice I have provided.

You may wonder why you never received the same information from your own doctor. From my own experience, I know how hard it can be for a doctor to dispense even the most basic information to all the patients who want and need it. Only too well do I remember one typical example of that difficulty. It occurred just before five o'clock on a busy afternoon. My desk was littered with the day's accumulation of paper: accident reports to be completed, patients' records, neglected correspondence — a full evening's work at the very least. And I was now precisely thirteen minutes late for a meeting with the senior professor of surgery at the university where I teach.

At that moment, however, I felt obliged to push both the professor and the paperwork into the back of my mind and focus full attention on the patient seated across the desk from me: a middle-aged woman who suffered from typical discogenic back pain.

Unfortunately, she was intent on telling me far more than I had time to hear. This was her first visit to my office, and she felt I should learn everything about her medical background. And so she went on. And on.

I fidgeted in my chair. I glanced at the clock. I pursed my lips as if I were about to utter something terribly profound about her condition. Perhaps that would cue her to stop talking and start listening. Would this medical saga never end?

At last it did. Concluding her narrative, she sat back in her chair and delivered one last, unforgettable comment.

"You know," she said, "I really appreciate this chance to sit and talk to you. The surgeon I used to see was always too busy. I'm so glad you have the time to sit and listen."

At that point I managed a wan smile but, as I saw her to the door, I realized, perhaps better than she did, that I had failed to give her the information she needed to control her pain. I had listened, but I had not advised. She would be back, and I would have to make time to add practical instruction to my moral support.

That woman's need for an empathetic ear and my increasingly heavy schedule provided the final part of my motivation to organize the groups that have grown to become the Canadian Back Institute.

As an orthopedic surgeon seeing a parade of sore backs day after day, I had found myself becoming increasingly bored with my own words as I delivered the same basic message to patient after patient. *Treat an acute attack with pain control movements and posture. Exercise to prevent the pain from coming back. Adopt good habits in your daily activities. Be patient. Persevere. Don't expect a cure, only control. Give your back the time it needs to get better.* Important and useful advice, and easy enough to dispense. But can you imagine having to say it over and over, a dozen times every day? Of course, there was a better way. I began educating my back patients in classes, usually groups of just a dozen or so, where participants, unlike my garrulous office visitor, have a ready-made, fully available audience: each other.

The concept of back schools was an idea whose time had come. My program rapidly expanded, becoming first the Toronto and then the Canadian Back Education

Units. Medical centers across North America, and as far away as Australia, recognized the importance of training common backache sufferers to cope with their own problem, and back education became the thing to do.

Our early classes were typical. You were invited to attend a series of ninety-minute lectures once a week for four weeks. Your first session was conducted by an orthopedic surgeon or other musculoskeletal specialist, who would outline the anatomy, physiology, and disorders accounting for common back pain. At the second session, a physiotherapist would describe the basis of physiotherapy and the effectiveness of back care, including exercise. A psychologist took over on the third evening, discussing the part that emotion plays in chronic pain and the behavioral aspects of back trouble. For the final session, you moved out of the lecture room and into an exercise room or gymnasium, where you could stretch out on the floor while the psychologist instructed you in relaxation and the physiotherapist reviewed good posture.

The purpose of our program was to give you a new appreciation of your back and its problems. Now you would have a good grasp of the basics, the same information I've set out in this book.

But we didn't win them all. At 6 p.m. one Friday, I got a call at my office from a woman who said she had just "failed" the course.

"What are you going to do for me now?" she demanded. As patiently as I could, I reviewed the highlights of what she had supposedly learned at the lectures. And then I threw the responsibility right back at her. What did she want to do next?

"What I really think will cure me," she said, blatantly ignoring the fundamental principle that nothing cures common backache, "is hydrotherapy."

Clearly, this woman didn't care to hear about the steps she would have to take to control her own back pain. It would not interest her to learn that hydrotherapy simply relieves symptoms temporarily. Since nothing else would do, I prescribed hydrotherapy for her — and made a note not to waste any more of the therapist's time, once that short program of treatment was finished.

My frustration with this response, both the patient's and my own, led to the creation of the Canadian Back Institute, successor to the Canadian Back Education Units. Working with dedicated physiotherapists, who believed as I did that the patient's active participation was essential for success, we opened the first CBI clinic. Our well-established education program was enhanced by a facility providing functional assessment and physical training. Here was an alternative to hydrotherapy and the other forms of short-term passive pain relief. Here was a chance for the patient to become involved; a chance to put into practice, under supervision, exercises and activities that could control the pain.

We will never be successful with everyone. But for every patient who wants only the easy answer and someone else to do the work, there are dozens who derive great benefit from the opportunity to talk honestly and openly about common backache and its control.

Anyone with an open-minded attitude can achieve an enormous sense of satisfaction from learning how to control back pain and from realizing that there is no longer any need to fear the next attack. And that satisfaction is somehow heightened when the learning takes place in a small and friendly group of fellow patients.

It's often said that misery loves company, but I am talking about a rapport that's warmer and far more humane than what the proverb implies. If you suffer from common backache, it is reassuring, to say the least, to realize that thousands of people right in your own community know exactly how you feel, and that others have absorbed the advice you are getting, have put it into practice, and have found themselves able to resume a normal lifestyle. The moral support that participants provide each other, almost from the beginning of the first lecture, is comparable to what occurs at a typical meeting of Alcoholics Anonymous.

That support has its practical aspects, too. One of my patients, a tiny woman I'll call Violet, complained during a visit to my office that she suffered back pain every time she drove her car. The car was an early-model Vega, with the brake and gas pedal set in an extremely recessed position. As she sat at the wheel, tiny Violet was forced to stretch both legs straight out — a position that inevitably arched her back and caused pain. I suggested that she have a mechanic modify the pedals, adding extensions or blocks that would permit her feet to be lower and closer to the car seat. She took my advice, and driving was no longer a painful experience.

Soon after that, she was attending a back education session when another woman in the class complained of back pain mainly when she drove her Vega.

"It's the gas pedal!" Violet cried, leaping out of her chair and bounding over to give her fellow sufferer the full benefit of her own expertise — where to have the pedals blocked, how much it would cost, even the name of the mechanic. Episodes like that make me believe that our students sometimes get almost as much satisfaction out of helping each other as they do out of helping themselves.

When attitudes like that prevail, the group's learning process gathers its own momentum. It's easier to accept and absorb new information and concepts when others around you are doing the same. Clients at the Canadian Back Institute quickly appreciate that they are there not to learn some cut-and-dried series of rote exercises but to understand their own spines and to use and strengthen them according to a set of simple, common-sense principles.

They quickly rid themselves of any notion of magical secrets and instant cures. They happily clear up all their old misconceptions about "slipped discs" and backs that "go out." They come to deal with back pain as they would a cut finger, giving it protection and rest while it heals, then getting it to move regardless of the lingering stiffness and pain. They gain a new appreciation of what their own doctors have tried to do for them. Usually they become better, more cooperative patients than they were before.

In that respect, I hope this book has the same effect on you as the Canadian Back Institute has on most of its clients. I hope you share their realization that you can take charge of your own back and its problems, and that in doing so, you will simply be following the example of thousands of other people who have problems exactly like yours.

Since you may never have the opportunity to make that discovery at CBI, I have compiled a list of questions that are often asked during our sessions, along with the answers you might hear.

Question: My doctor prescribed pills for me and I have been taking them. But you hardly ever mention pills. Don't you believe in medicine?

Answer: Certainly I believe in medicine — for people with diseases. But in the strictest sense of the term, you don't have a "medical" problem or a disease. You have a sore back that got that way from age and normal wear. It makes sense to take insulin for diabetes or digitalis for heart failure. Such drugs combat those diseases. But taking aspirin, or something far stronger, does not cure a bulging disc or a worn facet. Pain-killing pills, anti-inflammatory drugs, or even muscle relaxants may have a place in short-term pain control when they are combined with appropriate physical measures. They are not the first line of defense. They can't solve the problem. They should be employed when needed after education, counter-irritation, and exercise. Pills have no place in the long-term management of common backache.

Question: I realize I'm a little overweight. If I reduce, will my sore back get better?

Answer: Probably not, if you simply lose weight without adopting any positive back care habits. Extra weight is not a basic cause of back pain, but it does create two additional problems: it discourages you from doing the exercises that would help keep your back in shape, and it aggravates the pain caused by mechanical load. The degree of aggravation does not depend solely on the amount of excess weight unless you weigh over 300 pounds (135 kg). The pain is more closely related to body type, muscle tone, and where you put the added load. The tendency of men to put extra weight onto their midsections is especially pronounced. Women tend to add the weight lower and farther back, where it has little effect on the spine.

The tendency of obese men to have back trouble more readily than thin men was one of several interesting findings that came out of a study we made of more than three thousand patients at CBI — a large sample for a study of this kind.

Some of the other findings, in brief:

— Obese men with back problems tend to become even heavier as they grow older, while female back patients tend to become thinner.

— Tall people more often have back problems than short people.

— There are two periods in our lives when we are most vulnerable to common backache: between the ages of thirty-five and forty-five, and between fifty-five and fifty-nine.

— Women in their late fifties are the most vulnerable group of all.

Question: A few weeks ago I strained my back lifting a bag of groceries out of the trunk of my car. My back has bothered me ever since. What about accidents that cause this kind of back pain?

Answer: Major accidents are an obvious cause of back pain. People who sustain fractures of the spine will inevitably hurt, at least temporarily. But that is not the kind of accident that commonly triggers pain from normal wear. Only thirty to forty percent of people who develop symptoms from a worn disc or joint can relate the onset of their pain to a specific event or accident. Unless there is a need to demonstrate cause — in a compensation situation, for example — more than sixty percent of those suffering from common backache cannot identify the source of the attack.

Minor mishaps and even heavy lifting have nothing to do with causing or accelerating the natural aging process, although the strain may make the process painful for the first time.

To illustrate this point, I often use the analogy of the motorist driving a car with a worn tire. The car drives over a pothole and the tire blows out. What caused the blowout? If the tire had been new, it would have gone through the pothole without difficulty. If the worn tire had missed the pothole, it would have been good for another five thousand miles. Obviously, the blowout was caused by a combination of two factors — a degree of natural wear, plus a precipitating episode.

Question: I believe my back pain resulted from a pulled muscle, but my doctor told me I had a myofascial sprain. You haven't said anything about that.

Answer: Muscle sprains do occur in the back, but they are rare. Your back has a powerful group of small muscles that are well designed to protect themselves against damage. A significant injury, however, can harm the muscles in your back, just as a kick in the thigh can cause a charley horse. But it doesn't happen often, and it is not the kind of thing you experience without noticing it at the time. "Chronic" back muscle sprain is usually just a way of describing a muscle spasm that accompanies the mechanical problems in Pattern One or Pattern Two, and I've certainly said something about that. Generally, a "pulled muscle" is the result, not the cause, of the problem, and treating only the muscle pain misses the underlying condition, which can lead to more trouble in the future.

Incidentally, "myofascial" means relating to muscles and fibrous tissue. Myofascial sprain is just Doctor for a pulled muscle.

Question: You say that exercise is good for a bad back, but my doctor tells me to stay in bed. Who's right?

Answer: Prolonged bed rest, staying in bed for more than a day or two, has no value in managing common backache. Spending more time in bed can even be detrimental to your recovery since it weakens the muscles you need to get moving again. And bed rest in the wrong position can be just as painful as being on your feet. There is no role for bed rest in chronic back pain or for the patient with pain-focused behavior. For the acute attack, it's a matter of timing; do it early, do it right, but don't keep doing it.

Question: Should I wear a back brace? If so, for how long?

Answer: Use your back brace as you would a pair of work gloves — as something to be put on for a special purpose, then removed when the job is done. You wear work gloves when you dig in the garden, but not when you sit down to eat breakfast. If a back brace gives you a feeling of abdominal support and confidence during certain activities, by all means wear it. But loosen it or take it off when the situation no longer demands it. The brace is no guarantee against back injury, and its proper use includes good lifting techniques and a regular muscle-strengthening program for the trunk and abdomen.

Question: If I have a pinched nerve, can the nerve still function?

Answer: Yes, usually. Pattern Three or Four problems do not ordinarily prevent the affected nerve from functioning. Loss of normal nerve function, seen as genuine weakness in certain muscle groups or as an absent reflex, is rare. And remember, Pattern Three and Four are the least frequent causes of common backache.

Question: My exercises hurt. What's wrong? Should I keep them up?

Answer: If an exercise reproduces or increases your typical back or leg pain, don't do it. It won't harm you, but why suffer needlessly? There will be other exercises that are better at reducing your discomfort. Remember, we are talking about that old familiar pain, not the strain pain that accompanies any unaccustomed activity. It's reasonable to avoid anything that brings on your pain — unless it provides compensating benefits that constitute a worthwhile trade-off. Apply this principle to exercise, recreational sports, and any other optional activities.

Question: My doctor has told me I shouldn't wear high-heeled shoes because they are bad for my back. What do you think?

Answer: Shoes are never "bad" for your back in the sense that they can cause physical damage, but they can produce pain. Shoes with very high heels alter your normal posture, forcing you to arch your back in order to stand erect. If you have Pattern Two pain, that will increase your discomfort. So what it comes down to is this: each time you wear high heels, you are making another "withdrawal" from your "back account." If you are willing to accept backache as a consequence of wearing high heels, then my advice is to go ahead.

If you have Pattern One pain, high-heeled shoes can actually make your back feel better. I bought my first pair of cowboy boots from a salesman who had undergone a spinal fusion and who swore that the high heels on his boots were the only things that reduced his backache.

Incidentally, it isn't your back that takes the real punishment. Your body is so well designed that the effect of high-heeled shoes is dissipated first through your ankles, then through your knees and your hips, so that little of it reaches your back. In other words, high-heeled shoes put far greater stress on the bones of your feet and the muscles of your legs than on your spine.

Question: Are you sure physiotherapy is a good idea? I tried it once and it didn't help me a bit.

Answer: That's like saying you don't believe in "medicine" because you had some once and it didn't help you. There are many forms of treatment that fall under the heading of physiotherapy — hot packs, ultrasound, electrical stimulation, massage, and manipulation, as well as education and exercise training. If your doctor prescribes physiotherapy for you, ask him exactly what sort of treatment he is prescribing and what he hopes to achieve.

Question: How long is my back pain likely to last?

Answer: How long is a piece of string? There's no way to tell for sure. Each attack is the result of a number of separate factors, and the duration will depend upon the degree of wear in your back, your response to treatment, and your attitude, among other things. Separate attacks may run together, giving the impression of one continuous episode. As a general rule, however, an episode of Pattern One pain lasts from a few weeks to a few months. Pain in Pattern Two may be gone in a few days.

Question: Should I let my doctor x-ray me whenever he wants to, or is there some limit I should impose?

Answer: In the amounts medical doctors use them, and with today's sophisticated techniques, x-rays are safe. As long as your doctor knows roughly how many x-rays you have had, you should trust him not to overdo this type of investigation. But x-rays cannot see pain, and for the early diagnosis of ordinary mechanical backache, an x-ray is far less valuable than a good history and physical examination.

Question: What is the difference between a doctor, a chiropractor, and an osteopath?

Answer: A medical doctor holds a degree in medicine from a recognized medical school. Generally, his course is a four-year program following university, with an additional year or two of internship, a sort of apprentice period.

An osteopath is also trained in a four-year program, which includes many of the same elements as the standard medical school curriculum. Schools of osteopathic medicine are located mainly in the United States. The name "osteopath" suggests that these practitioners treat only diseases of the bone. In fact, they treat a wide range of medical problems, such as diabetes and high blood pressure. Osteopaths, like medical doctors, may attend postgraduate programs for training in surgery. Spinal surgery may be performed by either a medical doctor or an osteopath.

Chiropractors are trained in a four-year program that stresses spinal anatomy and manipulation of the spine. Their expertise is more limited than that of the doctor or the osteopath, and their treatments are related exclusively to problems that can be resolved by manipulation.

Question: Whenever I have an acute attack of back pain, the left side of my back swells up. What's going on?

Answer: What you feel is not swelling in the true sense; that is, it is not a collection of fluid under the skin. Your pain has caused your back to become very tight, and when the muscle is contracted, it appears to swell. Although in your back this is an involuntary action, it is otherwise the same as the muscular action that occurs in your upper arms when you strike the classic "strong man" pose by contracting your biceps. That is the likeliest explanation. Another possibility is that during that muscle spasm — a common response to back pain — your body is pulled over to one side. This posture causes you to stick one hip out, creating the impression that something has swollen up or "gone out of place."

Question: My doctor told me my problem is fibromyalgia. What is it?

Answer: The term "fibromyalgia" refers to pain associated with small painful lumps, which can be felt under the skin. They are found most commonly in the low back or in the neck or across the top of the shoulders. The lumps are a secondary condition related to the trigger points used in acupuncture. Certainly they are quite painful if they are pushed or squeezed. Fibromyalgia has never been shown to be a separate or primary condition. In my opinion, it is part of the larger problem of pain-focused behavior, an entity better described as Chronic Pain Syndrome. I think it is a mistake to give this one aspect of the condition a distinct identity. That makes it too easy for the patient and the physician to focus on a single physical feature while failing to recognize the bigger problem. It's like losing the forest for the trees.

The exact nature of fibrocytic nodules is puzzling; many surgeons have operated to remove the lumps, but when the skin has been opened, nothing has been found.

Your doctor may recommend that you have the lumps injected with a local anesthetic or cortisone. This can be quite effective in resolving the immediate problem. Even acupuncture needles inserted into these nodules can provide excellent temporary pain relief. Unfortunately, however, all such injections deal only with the result of a problem, not the primary cause, and the pain always returns. Even so, if you're the one who is in pain, you'd probably regard temporary relief as better than no relief at all. But to achieve a lasting solution, you need to address the far more difficult issue of chronic pain. You must face the circumstances that are the real reasons your pain won't stay away.

Question: What are the most important points for me to remember as a backache victim?

Answer: It would even pay you to memorize these:
— Back pain is not a disease and therefore it has no cure, but it can be controlled.
— Your pain is real — not just in your head.
— Emotional upsets can increase your pain.
— Some days will be better than others.
— With rest, posture correction, and appropriate pain control movements, your acute attack will subside.
— Back exercise is good — unless it reproduces your typical pain.
— "Hurt" and "harm" are not always the same thing.
— To make your back better, you need to spend the time, you need to have the patience, and you need to accept the responsibility.

Index

From Dr. Hamilton Hall, author of *The Back Doctor,* comes a remarkable book that can give you

Better Backs in 30 Days

Dr. Hamilton Hall, renowned authority on back ailments and author of *The Back Doctor,* presents a series of 21 exercises that will change the lives of most back sufferers in 30 days. Exercise, not inactivity or "rest", is the key to stronger, healthier backs. With Dr. Hall's exercise strategy, back pain can be avoided and alleviated, abdominal muscles trimmed, and posture and cardiovascular function improved.

This valuable illustrated guide can help eliminate back pain and the fear of temporary disability that often accompanies it.

SEAL

Seal Books

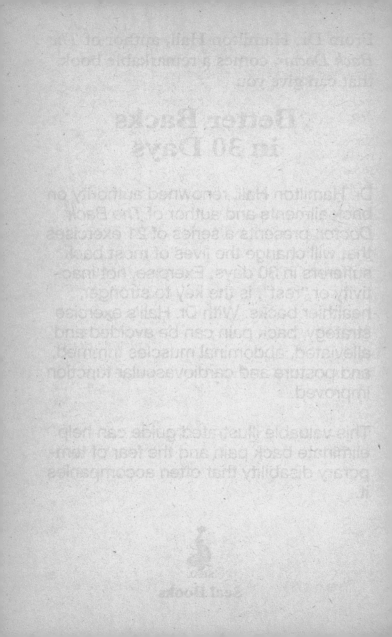

Seal Books

Offers you a list of outstanding fiction, non-fiction, and classics of Canadian literature in paperback by Canadian authors available at all good bookstores throughout Canada.

The New Back Doctor	*Hamilton Hall*
Never Cry Wolf	*Farley Mowat*
Ritual Abuse	*Kevin Marron*
Stories of Eva Luna	*Isabelle Allende*
Anne of Green Gables	*L. M. Montgomery*
Cat's Eye	*Margaret Atwood*
Born Naked	*Farley Mowat*
Lady Oracle	*Margaret Atwood*
And No Birds Sang	*Farley Mowat*
Butterbox Babies	*Bette Cahill*
Bluebeard's Egg	*Margaret Atwood*
Conspiracy of Brothers	*Mick Lowe*
Prized Possessions	*L. R. Wright*
Sea of Slaughter	*Farley Mowat*
Criminal Neglect	*Marshall & Barrett*
The Handmaid's Tale	*Margaret Atwood*
The Dog Who Wouldn't Be	*Farley Mowat*
The Crocodile Bird	*Ruth Rendell*
The Golden Road	*L. M. Montgomery*
The Suspect	*L. R. Wright*
Life After Billy	*Brian Vallée*
Hunting Humans	*Elliott Leyton*

SEAL

The Mark of Canadian Bestsellers